Dr Amanda Brown is a  ...ly prison in Europe, Bronzefield. She was a regular NHS GP for twenty years, until she gave up her practice to move into offender health. She has worked as a locum doctor in a variety of prisons over the past seventeen years including seven years in HMP Wormwood Scrubs, followed by six years in HMP Bronzefield where she continues to work to this day.

Also by Dr Amanda Brown

The Prison Doctor
The Prison Doctor: Women Inside

THE
PRISON
DOCTOR:
THE FINAL SENTENCE

Stories from inside a foreign national prison

DR AMANDA BROWN
WITH GUY ADAMS

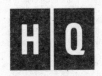

ONE PLACE. MANY STORIES

HQ
An imprint of HarperCollins*Publishers* Ltd
1 London Bridge Street
London SE1 9GF

www.harpercollins.co.uk

HarperCollins*Publishers*
1st Floor, Watermarque Building, Ringsend Road
Dublin 4, Ireland

This edition 2022

3
First published in Great Britain by
HQ, an imprint of HarperCollins*Publishers* Ltd 2019

ISBN 978-0-00-844801-1

MIX
Paper from
responsible sources
FSC™ C007454

This book is produced from independently certified FSC™ paper
to ensure responsible forest management.

For more information visit: www.harpercollins.co.uk/green

This book is set in 11.2/16 pt. Sabon by Type-it AS, Norway

Printed and Bound in the UK using 100% Renewable Electricity at
CPI Group (UK) Ltd, Croydon, CR0 4YY

This is a work of non-fiction, based on real events. Names and identifying characteristics
and details have been changed to protect the identity and privacy of individuals.

This book deals with difficult topics. The author has taken great lengths to ensure
the subject matter is dealt with in a compassionate and respectful way, but it may be
troubling for some readers. Discretion is advised.

This book is dedicated to my beloved husband,
David Martin Smith (10.11.1944–21.03.2021) whose love
and belief in me shaped my life, and who I have loved
with all my heart and soul for over forty years

Prologue

'I'm dead.'

The 'dead' man's name was Kofi Aboah and he was a giant. Over six foot of muscle, but shrinking. I could tell by his clothes that he had lost a lot of weight. His tracksuit slumped around him, looking as defeated as its inhabitant.

Most noticeable of all was a very large swelling on the left side of his neck.

I saw from his notes that he had advanced tonsillar cancer. *Too* advanced.

He had only recently transferred from HMP Wormwood Scrubs and this was the first time we'd met. This was not someone I could cure; all I could offer this man was kindness and the right to as much dignity and as little pain as possible.

In the yard outside, a delivery lorry was repeatedly warning anyone within earshot that it was reversing. In the waiting room two men were laughing long and hard. But it was as if those sounds were miles and miles away. Because in my room there was nothing but this 'dead' man and the photo of his family that he held in his hand. 'Dead,' he said again. 'My body just needs to catch up.'

He held up the photo so that I could see. Four people, his family, standing in front of their Ghanaian home, a rough-hewn brown hut on the outskirts of Tamale. The door was splintering, green skin rupturing to show sun-faded wooden bone, the thatch was threadbare. The ground all around them was a bright yellow sand. Just beyond their home a couple of women poked at the insides of a huge cooking pot with metal poles, as if whatever was cooking on this open fire needed fighting as well as heating. A small child, just apart from the cooks had noticed the camera and was staring longingly out at me, a character from a story that was just to one side of the one I was in. The family my patient wanted me to see seemed happy – happier, certainly, than this snapshot of their lives suggested they should be.

He turned the photo back towards himself and looked at it again. He had such an air of sadness about him. It washed over me and I couldn't help but be affected – a deep, bone-aching shiver of sympathy. My thoughts must have shown on my face because he glanced at me and then winced, as if embarrassed.

'Don't look like that,' he said. 'Not until you know what I have done. You might think I deserve it.'

'Nobody "deserves" to die,' I said, leaning back in my chair, which gave a little creak.

'Not even drug smugglers?' he asked, almost combative, as if daring me to disagree. 'I have seen all the expressions.' He smiled. 'The faces that start off sad, then become confused, become conflicted. I am used to it. Faces that change like the weather.'

'Nobody,' I insisted.

I understood the complexity of this man's feelings; he wasn't the first prison patient I'd dealt with who carried a sizeable weight of self-loathing. Some prisoners resented their sentences, some accepted them, and some felt they deserved even more.

He winced again as he shifted in the blue plastic chair next to my desk. His smooth head was shining with sweat, his left leg constantly twitching, up and down, up and down.

'You're in a lot of pain,' I said. It wasn't a question.

He nodded and looked down at the floor, as if ashamed. 'I tell them but they don't listen. Maybe they don't care.'

'That's not true either,' I told him. 'Nobody wants to see you suffer.'

'They do not have much choice.' His eyes moved back to the photograph.

'Your family?' I asked, encouraging him to talk, wanting to distract him. He nodded and, for a moment, his leg stopped twitching.

'My wife, Amba,' he said, pointing to the woman in front of that splintered, green front door. Her hair was in braids, tumbling in front of a slightly distracted smile. She wore a bright yellow and red dress, her arms stretched out as she tried to keep the youngest of her three children from running out of frame.

'She's beautiful,' I said, and he nodded in a matter-of-fact manner, accepting this not as an opinion but as a simple truth.

'She is perfect,' he said. 'More than I ever deserved. Much more.'

He winced yet again and his leg resumed its shaking.

'And your children?' I asked, still hoping to briefly distract him from his pain.

'They are perfect, too,' he said. 'Two boys and a girl.'

He pointed to the girl on the far right of the picture. She was fourteen or fifteen, beautiful but with such a tired look on her face. A young woman already exhausted by her life.

'Esi does a lot,' he said, as if having read my mind. 'Too much. She has to. With me not there … There is so much to do. There will always be so much to do.'

Outside, in the waiting area, the laughter had ceased, replaced by someone shouting, an explosion of foreign words that echoed and distorted to the point where I couldn't tell if they were expressing pain or anger. From experience it was probably both.

'This is Yooku,' said Kofi, pointing at the youngest of the boys, the one trying to escape the photograph and his mother's grasp. 'He always wants to be somewhere else. Usually chasing a ball. He is never so happy as when he's playing football. So much energy, so much power. The world seems too slow to him.' His face contorted with pain and I briefly put my hand on his arm and squeezed it very gently. 'It seems to move very quickly to me,' he said, teeth gritted. 'The days are so short and I am running out of time.'

I asked him about the treatment he had received for his cancer, but unfortunately, due to having been transferred to three different prisons prior to arriving at Huntercombe, he had never actually attended an appointment to get the treatment he needed. I saw the referral letters and appointments offered in the 'communications' section of his computerised notes, but he had yet to be assessed by the oncologist. I made a note to ensure he was referred as soon as possible.

But that didn't help him at that moment. He was clearly in a lot of pain.

'The first thing I need to do is sort out your medication,' I said, as I looked at his notes.

I saw that he was only on a low dose of co-codamol, and had only been receiving it twice a day instead of four times a day. No wonder he was suffering.

'How severe is the pain?' I asked. 'Does it come and go or is it there all the time?'

'It's always there, but then more pain comes and goes,' he said. 'So strong, so big … I've never known pain so big. It is really bad in my neck and left hip.'

A base level of pain coupled with breakthrough episodes. He certainly needed to be on stronger analgesia. Pain is subjective. Translating what a patient is experiencing and compensating accurately for it is always difficult, especially in prison where appeals for greater doses of medication were so commonplace they ran the risk of being ignored.

'I'm going to increase the dose and frequency of your painkillers, as well as try you on an anti-inflammatory pill with another to protect your stomach,' I told him. 'It should make a big difference towards you feeling more in control of your pain.'

'In control.' He sighed. 'That is not something I can imagine feeling again.' He gave a thin, weak smile. 'But thank you. You are very kind.'

'I'm also going to arrange some blood tests and refer you to the oncologist to see what treatment you need. I'll see you again next week so that I can adjust your medication further if needs be. There's no point in you suffering more than you have to.'

I sensed that for some strange reason he felt ashamed that he needed to accept stronger painkillers. That he was not man enough to just grin and bear it. He looked at me with such sad eyes and a brief silence fell between us. He felt so far away, beyond my reach.

Then the moment broke. He offered a small smile and held up the photo of his family again. He tapped at the final child in the photo. 'This is Kwame,' he said. 'He knows about suffering. He was born with a deformed spine. They tried to correct it but ... it hurts him to walk. Just to be.

Born into pain.' He looked at me. 'I sometimes think this is why I am here now,' he said. 'To suffer as he does.'

'You're not here to suffer,' I said. 'And you're certainly not here as punishment for your son!'

He sighed. 'Maybe you're right, I am just feeling ...' He shrugged. 'Just feeling.' He tucked the photo into his pocket. 'I am here because I smuggled twenty kilograms of cocaine into the country, that is all. And now I will die, alone. Here. That is that. I will never see them again. I cannot change that, I do not argue the fairness of it. I did what I did and now I pay for it. But my family are everything and I am not with them.' The fingers clutching the photo tightened and his arms shook, pain and emotion rushing through him. 'I have let them down. I have ruined everything.' He took a deep breath, trying to calm himself. His body slowly stopped shaking. And, finally, barely louder than a whisper, he said four more words. 'I shouldn't be here.'

*

'*I shouldn't be here.*'

I couldn't stop thinking about Kofi.

When I had finished the morning surgery I headed out into the waiting room and saw one of the officers, Alec. He usually worked nights so I didn't often see him but he was a really kind and caring man, one of the gentlest and quietest officers I've ever known. Years ago, when I had first begun working in prisons as a doctor, I had frequent cause to appreciate his kindness and support. I asked him about Kofi.

'There's no way he's getting out of here before he dies,' he said in his soft Welsh accent.

He was thin and pale in that way that a person working nights often seem to be, like an undersea creature developed in darkness and pressure. His hair was a rebellious salt and pepper thatch, never lying flat.

'That seems so wrong,' I said. 'Whatever he's done, he should be able to be with his family at the end.'

'You don't have to convince me, Doc,' he said, rubbing at a fringe that was reaching for the strip lights. 'He's no trouble, no danger; let him go home, that's what I say. The Home Office doesn't listen to me, though, more's the pity. He's got three years to go.'

'He really hasn't.'

'Well, no,' Alec sighed. 'But you know what I mean. '

'He doesn't seem the type,' I muttered.

'Type?' Alec asked.

I shook my head. 'Ignore me. I've been doing this job long enough now to know there's no such thing as a "type". I just can't picture him as a drug smuggler, that's all.'

'He says it's the first crime he has ever committed.' Alec shrugged, slightly self-consciously. 'And I know lots of them say that, but for what it's worth I believe him. He had a family, no prospects, and a ticking clock. He thought that the money would keep his family going after he's gone. Nothing else would. Not a choice I'd like to make.'

'No.'

I tried to imagine what I would do in Kofi's situation. Presented with an opportunity to set your family up after you've died, take away some of their worries, keep a roof over their heads. A legacy – one last big payday. Don't we all want our kids to be okay after we've gone?

'He should be sent home,' I said. 'It doesn't seem right.' Those final words again, stuck in a loop in my head. 'He shouldn't be here.'

'I know, Doc, I know.' We stood in silence for a moment before Alec said out loud what we both knew. 'Won't happen though.'

As I left the prison that day, stepping out under a darkening sky, I just couldn't get Kofi out of my mind. All patients are important, every single human being that passes through your care is a life that deserves your best attention and consideration. But, of course, there are always those who stick. Those souls who embed themselves. I couldn't stop thinking about him.

Kofi Aboah deserved to die with his family, and I would do everything I could to see that he did.

TWO WEEKS EARLIER

Chapter One

For a while the road is open. Green fields, stone walls, space everywhere. Then the trees close in and you're surrounded as you turn off, heading into the dark. Even the road breathes in, becoming too narrow for two cars to pass easily. On the right is Nuffield Place, one-time home of Lord Nuffield, inventor and engineer. It's a National Trust property, gardens to walk around, cream teas to be enjoyed. Further on is a care home. Prisoners of a different kind, perhaps – even the best solicitor in the world couldn't free you from your body.

The road becomes so enclosed, so completely removed from the sense of open countryside you've just left, that it feels like it was excavated, a tunnel cut through the trunks and branches. Of course, it might not feel so claustrophobic if you didn't know that, at any moment, you would see the sign for HMP Huntercombe. And, at that moment, the trees retreat to allow two large car parks and, squatting between them, the flat buildings of the prison.

During the Second World War this was a detention camp, its most famous resident – albeit only briefly – being Rudolf Hess. Few of those old buildings remain, but it still retains the low, functional look. Single-level buildings huddle behind tall fences. Red brick, tarmac and chain-link. Some prisons assert themselves, the dirty brown brick of Wandsworth, the huge functional walls of Belmarsh. Wormwood Scrubs more than most, with its famous towers and cream plaster decoration. Huntercombe is the very opposite; it doesn't draw attention. It doesn't impress or intimidate. It's just there to do its job in as flat and functional a way as possible.

I parked in the staff car park and looked across at the prison.

Huntercombe. Where my life as a prison doctor had begun nine years ago. From a GP's surgery to working as a prison doctor, initially treating young male offenders then moving on to Wormwood Scrubs, one of the largest and oldest prisons in the country and where I still worked three days a week.

It was an exciting and challenging life with every day bringing new difficulties, new faces, new purpose.

It had been three years since I had last stood there. So much had changed for me since then, but the place – at least to look at – appeared just the same. Looks were deceptive though, as had been made clear to me on the phone.

'The place has changed category,' the agency told me. 'You might find it quite difficult and different from any other prison you have worked in.'

'I'm sure I'll cope,' I replied, always reluctant to turn work away.

Life as a locum was never certain. So much of the work I did was – by its sheer nature – temporary. I was often covering annual holiday, sick leave, sometimes just working in a new prison for one or two days before I was gone again. This contract was two days a week for one year, covering maternity leave, which was good because it was long enough to become part of a team again, which was really appealing. I knew it would be hard but I lived with the knowledge that work could dry up at any time or I may become ill and unable to work, so I was determined to work as hard as I could while I was still able to. Also, even though my boys were grown up I still wanted to be able to help them if I needed to. This never-ending desire to support my family would take on chilling resonance, of course, once I'd met Kofi Aboah.

The air was cold and damp, that winter grey wetness that makes the grass fat and sodden and the sky heavy and close. I hoped my confidence about returning to Huntercombe would prove to be justified. After all, if I could handle working in the Scrubs, with all the drama and challenges it threw at me, then surely Huntercombe – however much it had changed – would have nothing too terrible for me to face? Even as I thought it, I knew I was being naïve. You can never assume anything about prison work; the next moment can always bring the very best or the very worst of life. But I wouldn't be facing any of it alone because, change or not, there were familiar faces there, old friends still walking the corridors from my first days there.

I thought back to the friends I'd made there before, the officers, the healthcare staff ... I am not sure if I would have coped with the transition from general practice to prison medicine without the support of so many wonderful people. And I was back for a reunion with some of those amazing people. Not least the Number One Governor, a man I knew well, who had taken up the position there only a few months ago. Indeed, it was him who had invited me to have a tour of the prison before my first day back, giving me a chance to familiarise myself with the changes before I started working there again.

I walked towards the front entrance, boot heels thudding on the wooden ramp. I pushed open the door and smiled through the thick glass of the security window in the gatehouse.

'Look who it is, back again! She can't stay away!'

And then, right away, the three years since I had last been there fell away at the sight of my first familiar face.

'Terry! Surely they have to let you go one day?' I said as I showed him my prison pass.

Terry smiled, his broad shoulders filling the security window. I tried to remember if I'd ever seen his legs. Try as I might, whenever I picture him it's behind glass, a grinning portrait whose good humour had greeted me on so many of my shifts.

'Never,' he laughed. 'I'm here for life. Didn't think we'd

see you back here though. You've been working at the Scrubs I hear?'

'I have.'

'Power to you,' he nodded. 'Can't be easy.'

'Is anywhere?'

'I suppose not,' he admitted. 'You know about all the changes here I suppose?'

I nodded. 'Prison for foreign nationals now. Rather different from the teenage boys I used to look after here'

'Eighty-odd different nationalities right now. Makes life interesting.'

'I bet it does.'

'Interesting is what gets us up in the morning,' said a voice behind me. 'Isn't that right, Doctor?'

I turned to see the governor walking towards me, the shiniest shoes in the prison service were now walking the corridors at Huntercombe, rather than at Wormwood Scrubs where I had last seen them.

'Hello, David!' I said, shaking his hand.

When I had first worked with David Redhouse, I'd been slightly intimidated by him. The sight of Shiny Shoes, as I had privately nicknamed him, marching towards me along the corridors of the Scrubs used to make my stomach churn with nerves. I had mistaken his professionalism and precision for coldness, which couldn't be further from the truth. Always immaculately dressed, he was a governor who made the job look the very last thing I imagined it to be: easy.

'Come through to my office,' he said, leading me away

from the security gate and off to the right, where a long corridor opened out into a handful of administration offices, including his.

'Have a seat,' he said, gesturing towards a meeting table at the centre of his office. 'Can I make you a coffee?'

'I'd love one,' I replied. 'Are you sure?' It felt very strange having the governor of the prison taking time out from his schedule to give me a tour, let alone putting the kettle on. 'I'm sure you must have more important things to do.'

'I cleared the time, don't worry,' he said. 'I'm all yours for now. That said, I'm also on my own today, so don't expect a miracle in a mug. It's me and a jar of instant.'

I gave in and sat at the meeting table while in the next room he clinked mugs, a kettle boiling with considerable enthusiasm. I looked around his office, a default screen saver of a non-descript beach became a Japanese garden. The walls were covered in charts and printouts; graphs plotted the year gone while calendars planned ahead. Statistics vied with projected targets. In the middle of it all, huge in a plain black frame, there was a black and white aerial photo of the place this prison used to be. Camp 020R as it was designated back then, the military detention centre.

'Here you go,' David said, bringing in the two drinks and sitting down opposite me. 'We'll have the tour first and then lunch if that's okay?'

'Lovely,' I said. There was a brilliant pub in the nearby village that always used to do great food. Beautiful old wooden-beamed corners and, with a bit of luck, a roaring fire. A return visit would be wonderful. A day of reassuring and comforting reunions!

'We'll grab a bite in the Rolls Inn,' he continued, referring to the café staffed by the prisoners. The name was a play on words, riffing off the term referring to when the prison roll call is correct and the 'Roll's in'. I tried to hide my disappointment. Possibly I didn't quite manage.

'The food is excellent,' he assured me. 'Cooked and served by prisoners under the supervision of a great tutor from the local college, a guy called Brian. They can end up with an NVQ in food preparation and cooking if they complete the course, so it can stand them in good stead for the future.'

'Oh … that sounds good.' I hoped the smile on my face was suitably broad. In all the years I had worked in prison I had very rarely eaten food cooked on site so, in fairness, it was another new experience and those are always welcome.

'What are the odds, eh? Finding you working here,' I said, changing the subject.

'It's very different from the Scrubs, and certainly offers a new set of challenges,' he admitted, taking a sip of his coffee. 'But I love working here.'

'Being governor in a foreign national prison must be like a totally different job though,' I said.

He gave a small shrug. 'The job rarely changes at heart: try to turn a few lives around. This place *is* quite the education though: the new languages, the cultures, the attitudes.'

'Not only with you but each other, I'd have thought.'

'There are a few petty rivalries between nationalities; you soon learn who doesn't play well with who. It's no different to learning the interactions between the gangs in other prisons. There are just a few more of them!'

Coffees finished, we got to our feet. 'Time for the tour?' I asked.

'Absolutely.'

David gestured for me to walk ahead as we made our way back towards the security gate. There, with a hiss, the barrier withdrew and David and I walked through in turn. He stepped into another small room housing cabinets of keys and, after placing his finger on the biometric scanner, the cabinet door sprung open and he removed a set of keys. I knew from experience that the cabinet door could only be open for a few seconds before an ear-piercing alarm would sound. The keys jangled as he clipped them to his key chain and then popped them into the leather pouch on his belt.

'So, what are the criteria for being sent here?' I asked as we walked out into the cold, winter air.

'In theory we only take people who are due to be deported,' David replied, leading me across a small court-yard to one of the wings. 'Foreign nationals who have committed a crime and are on the last stretch of their sentence come here before leaving the country. That makes for a very different type of prisoner. Drug problems are low, violence too ... These are people who have been through rehabilitation programmes before getting here.'

'What about self-harm?' I knew how much of a problem that was in every prison.

'We try to keep on top of it, of course,' he said, opening the metal door to the wing and then unlocking and ushering me through the heavy metal gate. 'And numbers are down, I'm pleased to say, but, yes, it can be more of a problem than some places. While the prisoners here tend to incline towards good behaviour, there's no doubting that many of the men are facing extremely challenging futures, and that's bound to express itself one way or another. Good morning, Mr Holland,' he said, greeting the officer on duty. 'Visitor for you. Doctor Brown, used to work here a few years ago.'

Officer Holland was a short man with bleached white hair, an off-cream dusting that hid tiny black roots. He smiled as we drew closer.

'Nice to meet you,' he said, shaking my hand. 'You're back here now?'

'I am.'

'Good luck,' he said with a wry smile.

'Now, now, Mr Holland,' said David. 'Let's not worry the good doctor. All well?'

'Quiet as you like,' Holland admitted, absent-mindedly plucking at his shirt front as if removing invisible hairs. 'Looked like Jacek was going to kick off earlier,' he added, 'but he's calmed down now.'

'Pleased to hear it. I take it he got his deportation date?'

Officer Holland sighed and nodded. 'December 20th.'

'Merry Christmas,' David said drily and sighed.

He led the way on to the wing. 'The constant issue here,' he said, 'is that many of the prisoners don't want to go back to the country they came from. Various reasons, either they don't see it as home – they've lived here in the UK for a long time, built up a new life and have friends and very often family here – or they know that they'll be going back to a regime that doesn't look favourably on them. Jacek is a case in point. He's gay and apparently that's becoming more uncomfortable to be in Poland. A good deal of public opinion is veering against same-sex relationships, I've been told.'

'And why would he want to go back to a country that doesn't approve of who he is?'

'Precisely. But, of course, it's not a simple matter to have the law take his side. His solicitor's been fighting to keep him here but he hasn't any of the official paperwork, no passport, and, right now, no choice. Of course, that may change, he may get a reprieve at the last minute. It happens.'

As our tour continued along the long corridors the air began to fill with the smell of cumin, coriander and chilli. Prisoners started queuing for food at the servery. I could see chicken wings, samosas, chips, a thick, dark sauce that gleamed beneath the hot lamps. It was already midday and the smell of food made me realise how hungry I was feeling.

'Governor.' One of the prisoners stepped over, his tray of curry and rice held out in front of him. For a minute I thought he meant to share his meal with David.

'Yes, Mr Malota, what can I do for you?'

Mr Malota had long, dark hair and a weathered face. He looked like he had spent a lifetime at sea, salt-blasted and cured. Just beneath one eye he had a faded teardrop tattoo.

'I need you to approve the visit to see my dad,' he said.

'Is the paperwork with me?' David asked.

The prisoner nodded. 'My solicitor says they sent it to you. You have to sign it or it won't happen.'

'I'll take a look, Mr Malota,' David replied calmly. 'Go and eat your lunch.'

'You'll sign it?' He raised his tray a few more inches, as if for emphasis, and a small trickle of rice fell from his plate.

'I'll take a look.' That David Redhouse control. Professional, polite and smiling, but unmoving. 'That's all I can say, isn't it, really?'

'I suppose so,' Mr Malota muttered. Then, with a defeated nod, he walked off, taking a cloud of enticing coriander and cumin with him.

'Mr Malota's father is in hospital,' David explained. 'It doesn't look good. Cancer.'

'Oh …'

'I'm sure we'll approve it.' David gestured for us to keep moving. 'But I can't promise as much without reviewing it properly.'

'Of course not.' I watched as we passed Mr Malota once more, settling down in his cell, the tray on his lap. He stared at his food as if wondering what to do with it.

'He's actually very well behaved,' David continued. 'Makes good byrek.'

'Byrek?'

'An Albanian pie … fine flaky pastry, layered with cheese, spinach and egg. Lovely. We have days where we celebrate some of the different cultures in here. People can cook some of their cuisine, maybe play a little music, bit of a dance.'

I laughed. 'I'm trying to imagine you joining in!'

He smiled. 'You haven't lived until you've polkaed in prison. The main rule we have is that if you want to attend your own cultural celebrations you have to bring someone who is from a different country. I like to think it spreads a little understanding.'

We kept walking through the wing, past a corridor of cells, prisoners of all nationalities becoming one in their grey, prison tracksuits. It was remarkably quiet, for a prison at least.

Perhaps David picked up on my thoughts.

'Generally, the population here is pretty good. They have their own problems, their own concerns, and I'd be lying if I said we didn't have disagreements from time to time – you know what prison is like … '

'I do.'

'But the behaviour in here is, for the most part, a little better than we've both been used to.'

'It's not the Scrubs?'

'Where is?'

He unlocked another heavy barred gate and swung it open. 'After you, Doctor.'

We stepped back out into the cold. A light drizzle of

rain had begun to fall as we crossed another courtyard and turned right towards a small, cheerfully decorated building. The windows were filled with posters, some handmade, brightly coloured collages, some more official, book covers promising everything from 'The Searing True Story of the Mexican Drug Cartels' to a hulking silhouette of fictional detective Alex Cross, his shoulders slumped in the murky, fog-bound world people like him always seem to inhabit.

'The library,' said David, pushing open the door, a smile on his face. 'The only escape we actively approve of.'

'Now look,' a voice immediately said as we entered the small building, 'you're going to complain about spending, but I used my own money for the last lot of postage so you're still winning and we should probably just call it quits, don't you think?'

A circle of easy chairs faced a cluttered desk. Rows of bookshelves asked for attention, puffed-up paperbacks, thumbed into a fan of well-read pages. Covers featured burly men weighed down by their own backstories and their maverick ways. A succession of mid-American skylines in various hues offered moody backdrops for Jack Reacher to stroll towards. Behind the desk an explosion of energy was shifting piles of books from one bit of rare space to another.

'Our head librarian,' said David. 'Asma.'

'Head librarian he says, like it's not just me and poor Julia who comes in on Tuesdays and Thursdays, and that's only to get some space from the demands of her cats. I mean … who do I boss about on any other day?'

'Me?' David asked, still smiling.

'That'll be the day.' Asma huffed and her fringe flew upwards like a permed windsock. 'Are you going to be annoying about my spending?'

'Am I ever?'

'You might be trying to lull me into a false sense of security. And you are?'

It took me a moment to realise Asma was now talking to me.

'Hi, I'm Amanda.' I walked towards the desk to shake her hand. 'I used to work here before it was recategorised. I've been persuaded to give it a go again.' Asma nodded as if she'd known this all along. 'David is kindly giving me a tour,' I continued, 'to let me see all the changes that have taken place.'

'Where will you be working?' Asma asked, narrowing her eyes slightly as if this were all very suspicious.

'In Healthcare.'

She nodded again as if all this were proof of everything she'd been thinking anyway. 'Are you a doctor?' She didn't wait for an answer. 'Very sensible thing to be,' she said, squeezing a pile of Terry Pratchetts to her chest, cheerful witches crumpling into folds of woolly jumper. 'My mother always wanted me to be a doctor.' She looked up towards the strip lights, as if remembering. 'I got as far as reading saucy novels about nurses before I realised it probably wasn't for me. I could handle the sauce but not the shifts.' Her gaze snapped right back to me. 'Not that it's much better here.'

'What is it you've been spending my money on, exactly?' asked David, sitting down in one of the armchairs.

'You said you weren't going to be annoying.' Asma found somewhere to pop the Pratchetts before turning her attention to a pile of cardboard folders overstuffed with dog-eared paperwork.

'Not annoying, just preparing myself. Accountancy isn't like a novel, Asma, I'd rather not be kept guessing until the very end. I want to know whodunnit.'

'And whatdunnit and how much it all cost,' Asma replied.

'Yes, yes. Just the Christmas cards.' She finally gave up on the notion of a tidy desk and put the folders back where they'd come from. 'The cards were mine, if you remember, but I'm not made of stamps.'

'Well, no,' David admitted. 'Of course not.'

'It's very important,' Asma said, having turned her attention back to me, 'keeping in touch with their families. It gives them a purpose. A reason to get their lives back on track. Some hope in, at times, an otherwise bleak world. Just knowing that someone out there cares about them gives them a reason to carry on.' She fell silent for a minute, lost again in her own thoughts.

'We do video calls, too,' said David. 'Some of the men in here haven't seen their family in years, it's quite something to give them the opportunity.'

'Video calls are a nightmare,' said Asma. 'Give me a cheap picture of a Robin and a stamp any day.'

David got to his feet. 'That certainly sounds more like

the sort of budget we have to work with,' he admitted. 'We must be getting on.'

'Do pop in when you have a moment,' Asma said to me, picking up the folders again in an inspiring refusal to give in. 'Not that you will have the time, but, well, it's nice to kid yourself now and then. Bye!' She carried the folders through a small door behind her and began committing acts of violence on an out-of-sight filing cabinet.

'Shall we?' asked David, gesturing towards a door on the other side of the library.

We headed through the door and into a corridor of small offices, where various people were sitting, heads down, sifting through paperwork and tapping at keyboards. Nobody looked up as we passed, lost to the constant turning cogs of bureaucracy that keep a prison functioning. Budgets and schedules, a constant balancing of cash and personnel.

The corridor opened out into a brick atrium. Through the windows I could see a handful of prisoners in tracksuits working a patch of garden. Thick bushes and low-growing winter vegetables, in regimented rows. One of them stood back and stared at the vegetables, admiring time well spent.

The atrium led to another corridor, this one lined with brightly coloured oil paintings. Bright blue seas splashed at orange lighthouses. Yellow tigers prowled jungles so green you might think the picture would glow after you'd turned the strip lights off.

'One of our residents,' said David. 'Swedish. He became obsessed with painting. Far be it from me to discourage him. Whatever keeps someone happy and peaceful.' He stopped for a moment to really scrutinise one of the pictures. It showed a horse with six legs galloping its way through a purple cornfield. 'We let him put them up on the walls. To encourage him, you know?'

I nodded, looking over David's shoulder and realising that the ears of corn had, well, ears. Fleshy lugs jutting out from kernel faces.

'Some of them are rather strange, it has to be said.' David scratched at his head. 'And he's taken to sneaking Swedish images into everything. African plains with little Vikings hiding behind a bush … ' He sighed, giving up on understanding what his eyes were telling him. 'Brightens the place up though.'

'Absolutely,' I agreed, determined to say something positive about the product of so many brush hours. 'Some of them are really good.'

'Some of them,' David agreed with a grin.

On the move again, he unlocked another gate and we walked through into yet another corridor – prison is nothing if not corridors and iron gates where a puffy West Indian man in a dog collar and sorry-for-itself suit was scribbling on a poster stuck to a wall.

'May I introduce you to one of our chaplains?' said David. 'We have a fair few, as you might imagine … Pastor Clive is Free Church.'

'Yes,' the man in the dog collar agreed, as if his faith had ever been in question, still scribbling away. His face then lit up with the most beautiful smile as he reached out to shake my hand. 'Good to meet you.'

'I'm not sure we should encourage graffiti,' said David.

'Absolutely,' Pastor Clive agreed, scratching at close-cropped hair that was thinning in the middle. 'It's the choir practice, you see.'

'Right,' David agreed, beckoning me to carry on past.

'Thursdays,' Pastor Clive muttered. 'Not Wednesdays, that's the problem. Poster's wrong. Not Wednesdays. Thursdays.'

'The men love Pastor Clive,' David said as we left the chaplain to his chores. 'He appears to be lost in his own world but has a heart of gold.'

We stopped outside a big pair of double doors. David pushed them wide and we stepped inside the gym. It was a large room, walls lined with parallel bars, equipment spaced out across the matted floor. Prisoners were pounding along on running machines, fiercely pedalling exercise bikes. In the far corner two men were lifting weights that made me feel tired just looking at them.

'It's an excellent gym,' said David. 'One of the best prison gyms I've seen, actually. I managed to wangle a bit extra on the budget.'

'I knew you were good,' I said, looking around in surprise, 'but not *that* good.'

There was never enough money. Nowhere near. That's one of the fixed rules of the prison service.

'I know,' he smiled. 'Sometimes I even impress myself.

The place is always busy, too. We even let some of the prisoners run classes. I have a guy from Poland who wants to go into personal training as a career. I'm only too happy to let him practise here. Isn't that what we're supposed to be doing, after all? Preparing these men for better, more constructive lives outside?'

'Absolutely.' I knew from past conversations how passionate David was about this. He possessed none of the fatalism I had sometimes seen in prison staff. He was a realist, certainly, but he was always determined to do everything he could to change the direction of the prisoners in his care.

'I'm trying to set up a programme where people who leave here share their successes with those still serving sentences,' he continued. 'Huntercombe Stories. We give the people who leave a card so that they can keep in touch, let us know how they're getting on, what they're up to. It's not got much uptake yet. Most people who leave prison just want to forget all about it, draw a line under it, but we have a few. People who've got a new sense of purpose, new careers. It does the men here good to hear about that, I think.' He nodded to himself and then gestured back towards the door. 'Well, enough of general prison life. Let's show you your office!'

We walked out of the gym and back the way we'd come.

'The man holding classes,' I asked, 'is that something he could get a qualification in?'

'Not from us, unfortunately,' David said. 'We do have education programmes, of course, prisoners can learn practical skills. As well as the NVQ in food preparation and cooking there's also a painting and decorating course, bricklaying too. We have a craft centre which we're thinking of turning into a shop. See if the prisoners can sell some of the things they make. Stuffed toys, jewellery, ornaments. All sorts of things. Even little hedgehog houses. Some of the men are very talented.'

'Hedgehog houses?' I asked, surprised.

'Yes,' David grinned. 'Isn't that what all shops sell?' he joked.

I laughed. 'Well, sounds good, you'll have to keep me out of there, though, I'm here to earn money not spend it!'

'Fair enough!'

We passed through another gate.

'Hello again, Pastor Clive,' said David. The chaplain had found another poster to alter.

'Choir practice,' he muttered as we went past.

'It's on Thursdays,' David called back, unlocking an iron gate and gesturing me through.

He led me to a final pair of double doors that opened out into the Healthcare department I remembered only too well. Very little had changed, the walls were still the same cobalt colour – though certainly it must have seen a fresh coat in the meantime. The waiting area still had its rows of blue plastic chairs, fixed to the floor – for obvious reasons: the behaviour might be better than in other prisons, but it made sense to minimise the risk of throwing chairs around in communal areas if a fight broke out, by fixing them to the floor.

Further seats were positioned along the corridor just outside the consulting rooms, where the prisoners would wait, hopefully patiently.

To my joy I saw another familiar face. Standing in the doorway of the consulting room, arms folded, ruddy face twisted into mock disapproval, was Rosemary Walbrook, one of the finest nurses I've ever been lucky enough to work with.

I first met her while covering for a doctor at HMP Reading not long before it closed. It was once the temporary residence of Oscar Wilde but a Young Offenders Institution when I had been there, just as Huntercombe had been. Rosemary was one of the most acerbic and yet, beneath all that, emotional nurses I'd ever known. I'd had no idea that she would be there, another familiar face to ease my transition.

'Oh my God,' she said, shaking her head as if presented with the worst news in the world. 'They told me they were getting another doctor in, but I didn't realise it was you!' She tried to suppress her magical smile. 'How am I going to put up with working with you again ... I'm not sure I can handle it!'

'Course you can,' I laughed, strolling over and giving her a big hug. 'That's what nurses are for, isn't it, putting up with people like me?'

'Absolutely!' Rosemary squeezed me hard. 'We're the real power here, and don't you forget it.'

'I'm sure you won't let her,' said David, with a smile.

I followed Rosemary into the consulting room I remembered so well.

It hadn't changed a bit: desk in the middle, lit by a view of the world outside through the barred windows, all sparse trees and condensation that day but strangely warm and welcoming.

'It's as if I never left,' I said.

'Your room may well be,' Rosemary replied, leading me back out and through to an entirely new admin block. 'But I know for a fact that this wasn't here when you last worked here.'

The new block was part of a wood-framed structure that had been added on to the original building, so the concrete floor was suddenly replaced with wood and a sense of the hollow space beneath. My boot heels thudded on the floor, and there was a disorientating sense of dislocation, as if the ground had become unreliable. It was like strolling across a kettle drum.

'We never did have enough space to work, in my day,' I said. 'You must be over the moon to have room to breathe.'

'We're rarely given much chance to do that,' said Rosemary with a smile. 'Now, are you going to keep cluttering up the place or can I get on with some actual work?' Rosemary pretended to look exasperated.

'I'll leave you to it,' I said, 'until tomorrow.'

'Don't be late!' She wrapped me up in another bear hug. 'Am I ever?'

And, with that hug, I suddenly found myself truly preparing to return to these corridors. Back to Huntercombe, so different and yet so familiar.

David and I made our way over to the Rolls Inn for our lunch. By then I was starving, and any sense of disappointment that lunch wouldn't be off the premises had been squashed. I ordered a kebab and salad which were really delicious.

After lunch, we headed back to the gatehouse, where he returned his keys to the cabinet before escorting me through the barrier and back to the outside world.

David stood with me on the threshold, looking out at a sky that threatened snow.

'It's difficult,' he said, after a moment, 'working here. But rewarding. You'll be fine.'

'Hope so,' I replied. 'We'll find out, won't we?'

He smiled. 'We will indeed. Wonderful to see you again, Doctor Brown.'

'Wonderful to see you too.' And with that, he went back inside and I made my slow way back to my little Mini.

I paused before climbing in, looking back at the building and remembering my nervousness the first time I'd seen the place. That sense of uncertainty as to what I was letting myself in for. I had a nagging feeling I was back in the same position again. Huntercombe had more lessons to teach me, I was quite sure of that. So many familiar faces, such unfamiliar situations, and a population that had the wide world of experiences, problems and stories to share with me.

It would be difficult – I couldn't guess how difficult, not then – but it would be a vital part of the next year of my life. And even on that first day, without having performed a single shift or consulted with a single patient, I knew somehow that it was exactly where I needed to be.

Chapter Two

REFLECTIONS

I shouldn't be here.

Those are the words, Kofi Aboah's words, that sunk into me so deeply during our first consultation. Why had they affected me so much? Why did they seem so familiar? So painful?

I shouldn't be here. It's a thought and a feeling that hangs miserably close in my life and has done since... Well, that's hard to say. Sometimes attitudes permeate so deeply they feel as essential as bones.

I think it really boils down to the fact that I have never really felt good enough. Maybe that's partly because I used to think that I must have been a disappointment to my father who I am sure was hoping for a son. My mother was too old to have any more children and so his hopes presumably evaporated when I was born.

I know I have so much to be grateful for. And I am. Deeply. And the idea of moaning or making a fuss is just not in my nature, but still, sometimes it's important to make a point. If there's one thing I've learnt in life, it's that you can't try and solve a problem until you try and understand what's caused it.

In 1982, a year after meeting David – a different David, naturally, not the governor of Huntercombe but rather the wonderful man I would go on to marry two years later – I spent a week's holiday with him on the Isle of Wight.

He was due to compete in Cowes Week, the oldest and biggest sailing regatta in the world. Hundreds of competitors take part with thousands of spectators gathering to watch. He was deeply passionate about sailing and participating in the regatta was one of the highlights of his year.

It was a beautifully warm summer and the atmosphere was somehow both balmy and electric as we walked along a jetty on the marina. We were admiring the beautiful yachts all moored alongside each other at the end of the day's racing, the wind making a haunted whistle through their masts, like a choir of ghosts.

We then took a walk along the High Street which was heaving with people all enjoying the wonderful carnival atmosphere, vibrant and throbbing.

Families with small children, groups of men and women carrying their kit back from the boats to their lodgings in bulging sailing bags, laughing and chatting about their day's racing. The pubs were all packed, people overflowing on to the streets. Children were running around with their faces painted as lions and dogs and tigers, some carrying colourful helium balloons that tugged in the breeze as they tried to fly away. Music from different bands filled the air. It was magical, and I was there with the man I loved.

We continued to the far end of the High Street, through the jostling, bustling crowds, as David wanted to show me where the guns were fired to start the races every day. They were located near to a very exclusive yacht club called The Royal Yacht Squadron. Membership was only permitted by invitation, followed by an extensive vetting and interview.

But as we passed by the gravel drive bordered by the beautifully manicured lawns that lead to the entrance of the yacht club, I noticed a sign that stopped me in my tracks: 'Dogs and women not allowed'

I was horrified ... The dogs got a better billing than the women, ranked in preference but still forbidden.

Although I was perfectly familiar with institutions that didn't want me, of course, as most women of my age were, it shocked and revolted me in equal measure and to this day I have never forgotten it.

When I was five years of age, we moved to a family home in Buckinghamshire that backed onto a beautiful golf course. My father was fanatical about golf and soon joined the club. I still clearly remember a sign outside one of the bar areas in the clubhouse saying 'men only,' which back then was so commonplace that I took it as normal. I grew up believing that women were second-class citizens and that I was inferior, but when I saw that sign twenty-two years later it was like being punched in the stomach.

My father was really keen for my sister and me to take up golf and asked us both one day if we would like to.

'No thanks,' my sister said, quick as lightning. She was a very good tennis player and had no interest in golf.

But I couldn't bear to let him down and so I agreed to give it a go, even though I didn't really want to.

I was twelve years of age at the time and my father tried his best to teach me the frustrating and deceptively difficult game.

I signed up as a junior member of Stoke Poges Golf club and we would regularly go to the practice ground where I would try my best to get the ball in the air!

Many years later my father and I used to enter the annual mixed foursomes knock-out competition. One year we actually managed to get to the finals and I don't think I have ever concentrated so hard on anything before or since as I did that day. To my overwhelming joy we won.

It ranks as one of the biggest achievements in my life and I was overjoyed that forever more I would have my name next to his on the winner's board.

Finally, I felt that I was no longer a disappointment to him.

I shouldn't be here.

Institutions that didn't naturally welcome women. Well, yes, I trained in one of those. A far more rigorous, stressful club. Women were allowed to study medicine, certainly, but I always felt that I had to try and exceed expectations to prove myself. I hoped that once I had qualified I wouldn't have to feel the need to justify my existence anymore.

I still remember the immediate thought that went through my head when I found out that I had passed my final medical exams. I searched in desperation to find my name on the list of successful candidates, and when at last I found it I was filled with the joyful thought that nobody could ever take this away from me.

In 1984 I was offered a job in a GP practice comprising six men.

'This is our token female,' one of the partners said when introducing me to the doctors at the neighbouring surgery.

I didn't take offence but just accepted it as par for the course at the time.

I shouldn't be here.

I'm not good enough

It's hard not to feel like an impostor sometimes when so often through my life I really thought that I was.

To never quite feel good enough, to feel unwelcome and that I didn't really belong.

It's hard not to think that, at any moment, I was going to get found out, challenged, ousted.

I shouldn't be here.

Yes ... those words affected me.

Chapter Three

HMP HUNTERCOMBE
6 DECEMBER 2013

Back I went, driving through the tunnel of trees to start my first proper day at Huntercombe. It was as cold as the day before, but almost impossibly bright. Crisp, frosted branches glistening, lawns laid out as carpets of light. When the sunlight blinked through the branches it was like a strobe light pulsing through the windscreen.

I parked the car and then walked gingerly to the gatehouse, holding a large cup of coffee I had bought at a petrol station on the way. This seemed like a good idea at the time. A nice coffee. Ready-made. Lovely. But walking across the car park I felt like I was in an egg and spoon race. The ground was thick with ice. I took tiny steps, worried I might come a cropper and end up with a twisted ankle and a scalded hand. My steps became bolder as I reached the salted safety of the entrance ramp, but, approaching the gatehouse, I could feel the anxiety levels gently rise about what the day would bring.

'Morning, Doc.' Terry was taking a drink out of a big mug with a dog's face on it. It made him look like he was about to bark.

'Morning, Terry, it's treacherous out there,' I said, relieved to see his friendly, welcoming smile.

'Yes, I know. I'll see if I can knock up some skis to help you get back to your car after your shift's finished. They're forecasting snow later on, so you might need them.' He beamed.

'Good man,' I replied, trying to hide my fear as I imagined a scary journey home. I was terrified of driving in snow.

I showed him my pass and he glanced at it before letting me in. The prison ritual: Terry knew it was me, pass or no pass, but I would always show it and he would always look. Because that's how security systems work. No exceptions, just rules. 'I'll call someone from Healthcare to come and collect you, Doc,' he said.

More rules, more systems. I wouldn't be permitted to draw keys and walk freely around the prison until I had undergone Huntercombe's key training again, and so to start off with I would need to be escorted everywhere. Regardless of how many other prisons I had worked in, or even the fact that I had already worked at Huntercombe, every prison requires its own key training to be undertaken before anyone is allowed to draw keys if they haven't worked there for a while. Frustrating, but a fact of prison life.

Just as Terry reached for the phone, a strapping Nigerian man wearing a nurse's uniform under his big overcoat, arrived behind me.

'Morning, Terry,' he said, holding up his pass.

'That's handy,' Terry replied. 'Doc, meet Abeo. Abeo, meet Doctor Brown.'

Abeo's face lit up with a smile. 'You're the new doctor?'

'I am!'

'Rosemary has told me all about you,' he replied.

'All good, I hope!' As if we ever really want to know …

'Abeo can take you over with him,' said Terry. 'Save you waiting around in the cold.'

'Of course,' agreed Abeo. 'Happy to.'

We passed through the security gate.

'Have a good day, Doc,' Terry called after us, returning his attention to his coffee. 'If you can!'

Abeo and I walked together to the Healthcare block chatting easily as if we had known each other for years.

'You were here before?' he asked. 'When it was young offenders?'

'Yes, my first time working as a doctor in prison. Straight from a quiet, cosy GP surgery.'

He laughed. 'That must have been quite the change! Young offenders …' He sighed and shook his head, smiling. 'I worked at Aylesbury for a while. Those kids could be … hard work.'

'How do you find it here?' I asked. 'Better?'

'In some ways, sure.'

Heading past the library I waved to Asma, who was framed in the window, wrestling with Mark Billingham – well, a poster for one of his books.

The smell of fried food was seeping from an air vent in one of the external walls, a white pillar of greasy steam escaping into the cold sky.

Abeo unlocked – and locked again – the gate and then the door leading to the Healthcare admin corridor. The business of locking and unlocking that is so much part of life when working in prisons.

We clonked along the hollow-sounding floor to the small kitchen area, where a number of people were chatting together. There was a lovely smell of coffee, and the room was warm and welcoming, especially as Rosemary was already there.

'Here she is!' Rosemary said moving forward to give me a hug. 'Here to get us all back on the straight and narrow.'

'Not sure I can promise that,' I laughed.

'Let me introduce you to everyone,' she said, pointing around the room, introducing each person in turn. 'This is Darren, one of our mental health nurses; Josephine, our long-suffering pharmacist; Shelley, who works in admin. Jake and Angela, two of our wonderful nurses, and Sam the lovely dentist who comes in twice a week.'

They all welcomed me and we chatted briefly. That all-important sense of family, of a team that worked together not only to help the patients but also each other. I glanced at the clock.

'Time to get settled in,' I said.

'I'll escort you,' said Rosemary, leading me out of the

admin block. She unlocked the gate at the far end of the corridor and, after locking it again, we walked along to the room I would be working in all day. Entertaining me all the way with tales of her new rescue dog, a particularly boisterous Yorkie named Maggie.

As she unlocked the door she smiled and said, 'Go get 'em, Doc.' And with that, she walked off, leaving me to it.

I stepped inside, turned on the light and settled myself down at the desk.

There was a Post-it note on the computer screen:

Welcome back, Doc. You'll be fine! xx

Good old Rosemary.

I logged on to the computer with my new password and looked at all the names on the morning and afternoon clinic lists, as well as the long list of medications that needed re-prescribing.

Fortunately, I was very familiar with the computer system they were using, so I also knew where to find the list of pathology results that would need checking and filing. I could see that the day was definitely going to be busy.

It was 8 a.m. and the clinic was due to start at 9 a.m., so I popped the lid off my coffee and set to work.

I began by reading through a small pile of hospital letters to check that they didn't require any action before being filed, and then started working through the list of repeat prescriptions.

Before I knew it, it was ten to nine and I could hear the sound of the prisoners arriving in the waiting area.

My first patients.

I could also hear the door of the treatment room next door being unlocked, followed by a gentle tap on the sliding door between the two rooms.

It slid open and an unfamiliar face poked her head around. She was petite and very pretty.

'Morning,' she said. 'I'm Saroj, one of the nurses. Just let me know if you need anything. I'll be working next door all morning.'

'That's great, thanks Saroj. I'm Amanda, be gentle with me on my first day!'

I was relieved to know someone was around if I stumbled across any problems.

Before calling the first patient in, I had a quick look at his notes and saw that he was 67 years of age and suffering from chronic kidney disease, diabetes and hypertension, all of which had only been diagnosed a few months ago.

I went to the door and looked out at the sea of faces staring back at me.

'Mr Holder?' I called. A man rose to his feet and walked along to my room.

He was astonishingly tall. I almost expected him to have to duck in order to enter my room.

'Hi I'm Dr Brown,' I said, gesturing for him to take a seat on the blue plastic chair next to my desk.

'I haven't seen you before,' he said in a lovely Jamaican accent. 'Are you new here?'

'Yes, it's my first day, so be gentle with me.' I smiled. 'How can I help you, Mr Holder?'

'It's headaches, Doctor Brown, the most terrible headaches.' He started rubbing at his scalp, almost unconsciously I felt, his palm sliding against his short grey hair. 'It's getting so I can't do anything. This pain, all the time.' Then, as if as an afterthought: 'And a cough. Dry and irritating, that's what you call it, isn't it?' He grinned. 'As opposed to wet and pleasing!'

'How long have you had the cough?'

He shrugged. 'Past few months, I reckon, but the headaches are what's really buggin' me.'

I continued to take a history, quickly realising that his cough and headaches were almost certainly a side effect of one of the medications he was taking.

'The enalapril you're on,' I explained, 'may be the cause of your cough and headaches and so it's worth trying an alternative treatment, which hopefully won't give you any side effects.'

'If you say so, Doc. I'll take whatever you give me.'

'I'm afraid you're overdue a blood test, too,' I said. 'Just to check your renal function and diabetes.'

He scowled. 'Can't say I like needles much,' he admitted. 'But if you're sure it's something I need to do?'

'I'm afraid so.' I tapped on the computer keyboard, booking him in with the nurse to have his blood taken. 'And I'll see you again a few weeks just to see how you're doing.'

As he stood up to leave, he looked so sad and wistful.

'It's kind of you to help me,' he said, 'but it all seems a bit of a waste of time really. When I get back to Jamaica, I won't be able to afford the medication I need, so what's the point? I'll end up not taking the pills anymore and then my kidneys will just give up on me ... and then what?' he asked, not really expecting an answer. 'Crazy,' he continued. 'Been here most of my life. I got a wife, three kids, seven grand-kids ... This is my home, you know? But they're gonna send me to Jamaica, where I got nothin' and won't get to see none of them.'

He looked past me out of the barred window, lost for a moment in his own thoughts. 'Makes no sense if you ask me. No sense at all.'

I struggled to think of something positive to say but fortunately he broke the silence, perhaps sensing how use-less I felt.

'Don't worry, there isn't an answer. I've spent enough time – days, weeks, years, trying to think of one.' He sighed. 'Thank you for seeing me, Doc. I'll see you again in a few weeks.'

He disappeared out of the door and I was left to wonder about what he said. I had to admit that all the effort in trying to improve his health problems would be in vain if he were soon to return to a country where he would not be able to afford the treatment he needed.

Accepting that a patient will often ignore advice and do as they please is one thing, but knowing that they were going into a situation where they would have no choice but to go against medical advice and treatment seemed ... Well, it seemed painfully futile.

The next prisoner was a much younger man in his late twenties. His name was Usama and I saw on his notes that he was from Syria and had a history of self-harm.

'Hi, Usama,' I said as he entered the room. 'Please come and sit down.'

He did so, quiet and gentle, as if afraid of making any kind of mark on the room or me. I noticed he was holding his arms in a stiff and strange fashion.

'Your arms?' I asked.

He nodded, slowly rolling up the sleeves of his tracksuit top. Each forearm was raw.

'How did that happen?' I asked.

'I cut them on anything sharp I can find,' he said. 'Anything ... even corners of brick walls can work. Then, when they scab, I pick at them to stop them healing.'

'And how does that make you feel?' I asked him. I knew enough about self-harming to know that the problem wasn't the cut – not ultimately – it was the deeper wound, whatever it was that kept driving Usama, and the many prisoners like him, to hurt himself.

'I don't know,' he said, staring out of the window over my shoulder.

For a moment we were both quiet. Then I decided to probe a little deeper.

'You're from Syria?'

He nodded.

'When did you come over here?'

He sighed and looked down at his lap. 'A couple of years ago. The fighting there ... you do not understand ... it is ... they shot the protesters. Do you know this? In Deraa. And the people ... they continue to protest, to demand an end to the regime of President Assad. When you protest here, in this country, with your signs and your songs, you do not expect tanks I think. Tanks and soldiers and bullets and death.'

He fell silent. I struggled for a moment to think of what to say.

'Yes, we're so lucky to be living in a country not torn apart by war,' I said eventually. What else could I say?

The civil war in Syria was likely to grow worse and worse. Usama would be far from the last to flee a country whose citizens could be tortured and shot for the slightest of suspicions.

'I ran away with Elias, my ...' he stopped, twisting slightly in his chair, awkward and uncomfortable. 'My friend,' he continued. 'But we got into some trouble. We crossed into Europe, made it as far as Chios.'

He looked at me, his eyes were so dead, a man who had lost so much. Yet his story came so easily from him. He was desperate to share it, desperate, perhaps, to be 'seen'.

'It is an island in Greece,' he continued. 'We met a group of people who wanted to get to Macedonia. A gang, smugglers, had made promises to them. A business, you know ... There are always people looking to make money by moving people around. We joined them. We paid. But the gang ... the money wasn't enough, they wanted us to smuggle drugs for them too. They said that if we did not, they would kill us.'

He looked at me, his eyes pink as he started to cry.

'That is how business is done in that world,' he continued. 'You make sure people have little choice. You make them say yes.' He looked out of the window again. 'Even so. We tried to run. People who act like that gang ... who can say what they will end up doing? Who can say if you survive after the drugs are delivered? So, yes, we ran. Elias and I, we tried to get free. Elias and I got separated. He ... He ...'

He shook his head, writhing in his seat, deeply uncomfortable.

'He was hurt?' I asked. 'Elias?'

Usama shrugged. 'I don't know. Hurt? Dead? I don't know. I never saw him again.'

It was clear that Elias had been more than just a friend. Something that, in Syria, would have marked both of them out as targets. Homosexuality was not remotely 'tolerated' in Syria.

I glanced at his notes. He was seeking asylum. Anything to save him from being sent back to a country that held nothing but death for him, both for his sexuality and because, at any given point, he could find himself on the wrong side of a wildly escalating fight between factions. And then it would be torture, beatings, execution.

I tried to imagine living with that. Fleeing a homeland

that wants you dead, never knowing if the person you loved, the one person you held onto to keep you sane, to give you hope, was alive or dead. I didn't have to imagine very hard: the result of such a life was sitting right there in front of me, raw in every sense.

I took a closer look at his arms, the flesh torn and ragged.

It all seemed so bleak that I wondered how I could possibly help him. I felt useless, desperately wracking my brain to think of how to offer him hope, but my thoughts were blank.

He was already taking antidepressants and was under the supervision of the mental health care team for counselling. So, with a heavy heart, in the end, all I felt I could offer was to try to show that I cared, and would be there to support him. I know that there are times in life when just being a friend to someone can help.

His cuts needed cleaning and dressing, so I stood up and slid back the door to the treatment room to ask Saroj if she was free to help him. Fortunately, she was, and so he shuffled next door to have his wounds patched up.

I was left trying to imagine how I would feel if I were in Usama's shoes, and as so often happened, especially since I'd been working in prisons, I felt overwhelming gratitude for my wonderful family and for the fact that I lived in a country that was not being ripped to shreds by war. The wounds that were really hurting Usama weren't on his arms. They were a distraction from the deep gnawing pain in his soul.

Two patients in, and I felt that I couldn't really help

either of them. Not in any way that would actually last. Not in a way that felt like anything more than a sticking plaster.

The next patient on my list was a man in his mid-forties called Serge Wemba. He was medium height with short, cropped hair and kind twinkly eyes.

'Doctor!' he said, as if we were old friends finally reunited.

'Hello' I said, as he sat down. 'Pleased to meet you. So, Mr Wemba, what can I do for you today?'

'Well, Miss,' he replied, in a thick south London accent, 'I got these really itchy feet, and they're drivin' me mad!'

With that he took off his shoes and started peeling off his smelly socks.

'Sorry about the smell,' he said looking slightly embarrassed.

'I've smelt much worse,' I replied with a smile. 'Tell me, what's your story, Serge? Will you be going home soon?'

As soon as I'd spoken, I realised that it was, perhaps, not the most sensible question to lead with.

'Sending me home? They're not sending me home! They're sending me to the Congo! I can't even speak French! What am I supposed to do in the bloody Congo, mate? I've got no family there, no friends, no chance. It's crazy. They're gonna send me somewhere I don't even remember.'

'You were born there?'

'Yeah, but I've been living in Brixton since I was a kid. You want to send me home? Then send me to Windmill Gardens!'

He looked confused for a moment, as if trying to imagine how he was going to cope living in a country that was so far removed from the world he knew.

'Congo,' he said. 'I ask you.' He looked at me, a slightly cheeky look in his eyes. 'You know what the capital is?'

'Of the Democratic Republic of Congo?' Oh dear ... I was so embarrassed. 'Erm ...'

He laughed. 'There you go, see? Who knows? I mean, I do, 'cos I googled the sod, didn't I? Looked it up. Kinshasa. Biggest city in Africa. Fifteen million people. That's nearly twice the population of London, innit? And they're going to dump me right in the middle of the bastards. Number fifteen million and one. There you go, Serge. 'Ave at it.'

He shook his head, as if it were all the most stupid thing he had ever heard. Then, with a sigh, he slumped in his seat, the fight gone from him for now.

'Well, Doc,' he said, 'I tell you. I got these itchy feet, yeah? They're just too much for me to stand, driving me nuts. What can you do for 'em?'

I checked his feet and it was clear that he had a fungal infection.

'I'll prescribe a really good antifungal cream for you, which you can collect from the pharmacy later today. Dry your feet thoroughly and use the cream twice a day. The infection should clear up nicely.'

He nodded, deflated but doing his best to hold it together. 'See? One thing at a time. That's the way.'

He got to his feet. 'Thanks, Doc, sorry to have a rant, not your fault.'

He walked out.

As the morning wore on the theme was fairly consistent. Awful story after awful story, people from all over the world who had now washed up in HMP Huntercombe ... I was used to patients in prison being very forthcoming, they frequently took the opportunity to engage with someone new, to share a little of themselves, but here it was even more pronounced. So many people desperate to speak, to let out all their frustrations.

I stood at the window for a few moments, just to put a comma into the long stretch of the morning so far. A few flakes of snow were gently falling, and I reflected on all the people I had met that day. My thoughts were interrupted by a gentle knock on the door.

'Come in,' I called.

The door opened and I turned to see a man in his late thirties.

'Is it okay to come in?' he asked. 'I have an appointment at 11.30.'

'Yes, of course.' I beckoned him towards the chair and sat back down at my desk. 'Let me just get your notes up on the computer, bear with me.'

I clicked on the next name on the appointment ledger.

'Mr Kobe?'

'Yes, Daniel Kobe.'

A wide smile lit up his wonderfully friendly face.

'I haven't seen you before, have I?' he asked.

'No, it's my first day.'

'Well, there's a thing, it's nearly my last.'

I must have appeared worried as I looked at his notes on the computer, because he immediately qualified his statement.

'Not in life!' he laughed. 'I'm here because I have sprained my wrist – nobody ever died of a sprained wrist.' He held up his left hand and waved it slowly. 'I mean one of my last days in this prison. They are sending me home.'

Home? That was the last place most of the prisoners seemed to feel they were going.

'Where's home for you, Daniel?'

'Ghana! I'm going back to Ghana.' He laughed then gave a huge, theatrical shiver. 'I can't wait. Just look out of that window. It is colder here than in an evil man's heart, don't you think? I cannot wait to be back in a country that knows what warmth is.'

'You're happy to go, then?'

'Happy? I am over the moon!' He lowered his voice in mock secrecy. 'They even pay for your flight, you know. Can't be bad, eh?'

'That's really wonderful to hear,' I said. Daniel's enthusiasm couldn't quite outweigh the darkness of the rest of the morning, but I was relieved to meet someone who was happy with what the future held for them.

I leaned forward. 'Can I have a look at your wrist?'

'Of course.' He held out his arm. 'I injured it in the gym a few days ago.'

He sucked air in through his teeth as I gently touched his wrist to check that there was no sign of a scaphoid injury. One of the small bones in the wrist, it can lead to problems long-term if a break isn't diagnosed and dealt with. Happily, there was no suggestion of anything more serious than a sprain, so his self-diagnosis was perfectly correct.

'A compression bandage and some anti-inflammatories will do the trick,' I said.

'Pills?' he asked. 'Do I have to? I hate taking pills. Try to avoid it if I can.'

'Okay. I can prescribe anti-inflammatory gel instead, if you prefer? Just rub it in three times a day and with time and rest it should soon settle down.'

'Perfect.' He got to his feet. 'First day, eh? Well, I hope you enjoy working here. It's not all bad!'

'I'm sure it's not.'

'I envy you,' he said, walking back towards the door. 'I'm longing to work again. I have had far too much time to dwell on things, locked up in here. It's not healthy.' He stopped in the doorway. 'An empty mind is the Devil's workshop,' he said. 'That's what they say, isn't it, Doctor Brown? I think that's so true. Thanks for seeing me.'

'You're welcome, Daniel. Good luck with your new life.'

'I'll make it a busy one,' he replied, nodding, then, with a smile, he stepped out of the consulting room.

The Devil's workshop. I've spent plenty of time in there over the years. Most of us have, left with our own thoughts and fears, the very worst bouncing around our heads in those moments when there's nothing else to distract or occupy us.

I thought about the rest of the prisoners there, many of them trapped somewhere far smaller than their cell. Look at poor Usama, constantly trying to get out of the numb, horror-filled box of his own memories. When he cut his arms, it wasn't his arms he wanted to tear open, it was likely himself. To feel, to understand, to move on and finally heal.

The Devil's workshop. Yes. I could already see that many of my patients would be suffering from the effects of spending time there. My job, as was so often the case, wouldn't be so simple as trying to help their bodies. Their minds would be where the biggest wounds lay.

Chapter Four

It had been three weeks since I had returned to work at Huntercombe. Finally, having completed my key training, I was free to move around the prison without needing to be escorted. I was also no longer in the slightly humiliating position of having to ask to have the loo unlocked every time I needed to use it, knowing that someone had to wait outside to lock it up again when I had finished. Much easier.

In many ways it felt like a lot longer than three weeks. I had met such a variety of patients in that time, each with their own stories, with their own problems, with their own fears. And, of course, Kofi Aboah that gently spoken giant, clutching a photograph of his family, knowing that he was dying and that time was running out.

I realised that there was probably very little that could be done, but I was determined to try. I would do all I could to find out if there might be a way of helping him to be released early, on compassionate grounds, and to return him home to end his days surrounded by his family.

Making the usual brief walk between my car and the gatehouse, I decided that I would find the time that day, if possible, to dig into Kofi's situation a little deeper. There was absolutely nothing to be lost in trying to help.

As I was approaching the gatehouse, I saw Terry standing in the entrance beckoning to me.

'Good timing, Doc!' he called. 'Get your skates on, we need you.'

It's lovely to be needed, but hearing that, as a doctor, more often than not made my blood run cold.

I broke into a jog up the entrance ramp, my heart rate notching up a level. Adrenalin levels rising.

'What's the problem?' I asked, worried about the answer I was about to hear

'One of the prisoners,' said Terry. 'In a bad state, got the officers in a panic.'

I flashed my pass at him – even at times like those, the rules must stand, perhaps especially so. Emergencies can be when mistakes happen – adrenaline pumping, the clock ticking, and yet that's when everyone needs to be even more careful.

Terry went back inside his office to open the security panels and let me through. I noticed David Redhouse striding at speed down the corridor towards me.

'Good timing,' he said as he gestured for me to go ahead.

We both buzzed out a set of keys in turn and clipped them on to our key chains.

'I assume Terry told you about the patient on Mountbatten,' David said, both of us jogging now. 'I was just on my way to find out what's going on, but I must admit to being relieved that you're here to accompany me.' He opened the gate and we stepped outside.

'Is there anything you can tell me as we go?' I asked.

'Young man's name is Akeem Grace, 27 years of age. According to the officer he has very severe abdominal pain, diarrhoea and vomiting.'

'And he's the only one?' I asked, trying to keep up. 'Nobody else has the same symptoms?'

'No,' he replied with a half-smile. 'I am very pleased to report that he's the only one. I trust you weren't going to cast aspersions towards the catering staff?'

'Never.' I returned the half-smile. 'Just checking.'

I opened the gate to Mountbatten Unit, and ushered David inside. I saw Saroj following right behind us.

'I'll lock the gate' she shouted. 'You carry on.'

The entrance corridor opened out to a small common area with a pool table, beyond which was the corridor of cells. I could see an officer I didn't know standing at the far end, hovering nervously outside the open door of the prisoner's cell.

'It's all right, Mr Thomson,' said David. 'Help is at hand. You can breathe out now.'

Saroj came jogging up to us and David stepped back,

allowing us to both step inside the cell. The overpowering smell of sickness, sweat and diarrhoea felt as if it actually hit me in the face. It was hot and pungent, making the room feel even more claustrophobic than it normally would.

'Hello, Mr Grace,' I said, moving over to the prisoner who was lying on the bed. His face was covered with sweat, his eyes barely focusing as he looked towards me. His breathing was rapid and he was wheezing, as if he was struggling for air.

'I'm Doctor Brown,' I told him, 'and you may well know Saroj. Is it okay if we examine you?'

For a moment it was as if he hadn't heard us, those unfocused eyes glazing for a second before moving back towards me.

'Mr Grace?' I asked again.

He nodded his agreement, and so Saroj proceeded to quickly check his sugar level and oxygen saturation, both of which were normal. His temperature, however, was raised at 38.5.

'Can you pop your tongue out for me?'

His movements were sluggish, but he slowly protruded his tongue. The briefest glance showed that it was dry, which was hardly surprising as he was likely to be dehydrated after all the diarrhoea and vomiting.

'Do you have any medical conditions I should be aware of, Mr Grace?' I asked. 'Are you on any medication currently?'

His eyes kept glazing over; he obviously wasn't able

to concentrate sufficiently to help me with any clear answers. I listened to his chest and heard a few minor crackles and scattered wheezes.

'Do you know if Akeem has a history of asthma, Saroj?' I asked.

'Certainly not that we're aware of,' she said, looking puzzled. 'He's normally very fit and well. Never gives us any trouble.'

'Can you tell me where it hurts, Mr Grace?' I asked, but he just groaned.

I started to gently press on his abdomen, which was mildly tender all over, but a little more so in the lower right-hand side, raising the possibility of appendicitis.

He was clearly far too unwell to remain in prison, and needed to be admitted to hospital, and although appendicitis was high on the list of possible diagnoses, I have been caught out far too many times over far too many years to be certain of it. At least there was no sign of the particular tenderness or tension that could suggest peritonitis, which was certainly good news.

I braced myself to go to report back to David. It felt a bit like déjà vu from my previous encounter with him in Wormwood Scrubs, some while ago. Back then, my insistence that a prisoner be admitted to hospital had caused considerable distress and concern (though, in the end, it had been proven only too necessary). This time I think David was expecting it. I stepped outside the cell.

'I'm sorry but he definitely needs to go to hospital,' I said.

Rather than his expression changing to one of exasperation and frustration, as it had last time, he just sighed.

'It's the Scrubs all over again is it?' he said, almost smiling. 'Oh well. Better get organised. What do you think is wrong with him?'

'It might be appendicitis,' I replied. 'But I can't be absolutely certain with a limited history. He'll have to have blood tests, most likely a chest X-ray, abdominal scans, and whatever else the hospital doctors decide that he may need.'

David nodded. 'Right. Well, Mr Thomson, can you arrange the ambulance and sort out all the paperwork?'

'Thank you, David,' I said, feeling so relieved to know that help would soon be on its way. 'Might I be able to speak with you later?' I asked. 'Maybe in my lunch break? It's about Mr Aboah.'

'Yes, of course,' he said. 'That should be okay. I'm usually free between half twelve and one, if that suits you?'

'I'll do my best,' I said, because I never quite knew what prison might throw at me to scupper my plans. 'Thank you so much.'

I went back into Akeem's cell to explain that we were arranging for him to go to hospital. Although normally a prisoner would not be informed of an impending hospital attendance, in this case I was fully aware that Akeem would be supervised by an officer at all times until the ambulance arrived and felt it only right to let him know that help was on its way. Besides, it was clear from the state he was in that he wasn't about to plan an escape. He was far too ill to attempt any such thing.

Saroj and I walked back to Healthcare together as it was nearly time for me to start my clinic.

'How are you finding it here?' she asked.

'Disheartening at times,' I admitted. 'I'm afraid I sometimes find it hard to accept that the help I can offer is often quite limited because of the stress so many of the men are under due to the uncertain futures they are facing'

She nodded. 'Yes. Like poor Usama.'

'Ah, yes,' I said, thinking of the tragic young Syrian man. Saroj would have cleaned up his wounded arms many times, I was sure. 'Poor Usama indeed.'

As we entered Healthcare, I was surprised to see Daniel Kobe standing in the corridor with a mop and bucket.

'Mr Kobe?' I said. 'Shouldn't you be in Ghana? What's happened?'

'Yes, Dr Brown,' he replied with a huge smile. 'Ghana is exactly where I should be! Exactly! But instead, there is a problem with paperwork and my lawyer is talking to another lawyer and … Oh, who knows what is going on? I'm not too worried though, as I have been assured that it will all get sorted soon. That is what the lawyers all say. They use the word "soon". Do you want to know what I think about that word, doctor?'

'I do.'

'I do not think it means what lawyers think it means.'

'I understand.'

'So, all I do know with any surety is that I am still here.'

'With a mop.'

'With a mop. Because an empty mind is the Devil's workshop, remember?'

'I certainly do. I really related to that when you told me,' I admitted.

'I could see,' he replied, nodding and tapping at his temple. 'You are one who knows that workshop, I think. And I feel lucky to have been given a job at long last. I have been asking for a while but it's finally happened, and here I am, the Healthcare cleaner.'

He stepped back and, swinging the mop and bucket to one side, bowed low.

'That's great. Wonderful to hear some good news. We're lucky to have you.'

'I know,' he said with a cheeky grin. 'I will keep your room tidy and your floor sparkling.'

'I'm sure you will. How's the wrist by the way?'

'Healed perfectly, thanks to my excellent doctor.' He grinned as he spun his mop in the bucket of soapy water again. 'Just look at that. There's nothing I can't do.'

'Very impressive!' I said, smiling. I started towards my room but stopped as a thought suddenly occurred to me. 'Mr Kobe?'

'Oh please, call me Daniel, Miss.'

'Daniel it is. Do you know someone by the name of Kofi Aboah? He's from Ghana, too.'

'Really? I don't think I do. Which is strange, as I thought I knew all the people here from God's own country.'

'He's not been here very long, and I think he's feeling a bit lost and lonely. He probably keeps himself to himself. Still, I'm sure it might help if he met a few friendly people from his home country. A few friendly faces, you know?'

'I have the friendliest face in the whole prison! You know this! Leave it with me and I will look out for him. I'll get him to meet my friends and they will introduce him to their friends. I'm sure between us we will manage to make sure he knows everyone.' He gave me a final, completely sincere smile. 'Don't worry, Doctor Brown, I will do my very best to make him happy for you.'

I wasn't sure anyone but his family could do that, but I was relieved to know that Daniel would be looking out for him too. A man like Kofi couldn't have too many people on his side. He needed all the support he could get.

'I would appreciate any help you can give him, Daniel,' I said. 'He's a good man and he misses his family very much.'

'And the sunshine, Doctor, never forget the sunshine.' Daniel leaned in as if sharing a secret. 'You know, this morning it was two degrees Celsius out there. Two. How can anyone survive in such a freezing country? We may as well all try to get by on the moon.' He laughed, pleased with this absurd idea and shuffled off, wheeling his mop bucket in front of him. The wheels of the bucket squeaked loudly, as if giggling right along with him.

'Morning,' came a voice from behind me. It was Darren, one of the mental health nurses. He was a young man, extremely tall and thin. It wouldn't have been that hard to pick him up and dunk his feet in Daniel's mop bucket. He always wore a stubble beard, pale chin covered in iron-filings. In his left ear he had a large piercing that made me think of a wine stopper, a silver ball on one end, a gleaming cone on the other.

'How are you this morning?' he asked.

He had a soft Lancashire accent and always spoke so quietly that, at times, when the prison was at its noisiest – and prisons can be very noisy indeed – I had to strain to hear him.

'Not the best start,' I admitted, and told him about Akeem.

He scratched nervously at his stubble at the thought of Akeem's pain.

'Well done on getting him to the hospital,' he said. 'I'm sure they'll get to the bottom of it.'

'Yes,' I agreed, 'once he's had a few tests done.'

'I spoke to one of your patients yesterday,' said Darren. 'Usama Hassan? The poor young man who fled Syria, losing his partner on the way. Do you remember him?'

'Of course, I do. Has he been self-harming again?' I asked, knowing only too well how likely that was. It could be very difficult to change such patterns of behaviour. Mental illness is rarely straightforward and can be so unpredictable and hard to fathom at times. *The Devil's workshop*, I thought.

Darren nodded. 'I got Rosemary to patch him up. But we had a good talk. I'm hopeful we can get through to him.'

'I hope so, he was in such pain.'

'Yes,' Darren nodded, and began nervously fiddling with his piercing. 'He spoke highly of you, by the way.'

'That's nice to hear,' I told him. 'But I didn't do anything special; it'll be you that makes the difference, I'm sure.'

He shrugged. 'It's a group effort. We're all just doing our best.'

'We are,' I agreed. 'And on the subject of which, I need to get started.'

'Of course,' he agreed, looking around and, seemingly, only just noticing that patients had begun to appear. 'Yes,' he nodded again, as if understanding finally. 'Busy, busy.'

'Always,' I agreed, saying goodbye and heading towards the consultation room, wondering what the rest of the day had in store.

*

My first patient, Habib Khan, presented one hugely awkward problem the moment he wrestled his way through the door and into the room.

'Oh,' he said, looking at the plastic bucket chair. 'Now, you see, it's like this, two things might happen if I try to sit in that. One: I end up wearing it for the rest of the day. Or, two: I break your chair and we will then both have to deal with the most awkward business of me lying on your floor.' He looked at me, his eyes twinkling. 'And we do not want that, learned Doctor Brown, it would be horrid for us both.'

Mr Khan was – as his notes confirmed – two hundred and thirty-four kilos, just shy of thirty-seven stone. And, with some embarrassment, I realised he may well be right; the chair would likely not accommodate him. For a second I was at a loss as to what to do, but then it occurred to me that some of the chairs in admin were a bit more robust, with padded seats.

'It's definitely not the most comfortable seat in the world,' I said with a smile, getting to my feet and moving past him to the door. 'So just step outside for a moment while I try to find you a better one.' He nodded and shuffled back out into the waiting room. I locked the door and walked along the corridor to the admin block.

As quickly as possible, I managed to find a more substantial-looking chair and wheeled it back to my room. Mr Khan followed me back in and I did my very best not to look nervous as he slowly, and with some effort, lowered himself down into it.

'That,' he said, safely supported, 'is a relief to us all and, if I might say, the end to a particularly embarrassing start to this consultation.'

'Please,' I said, back behind my desk and looking at his notes on the computer. 'There's no need to be embarrassed, the fault is with the furniture. What can I do for you today, Mr Khan?'

'Well, the good news is that I am finally on a diet!' he grinned. 'Which is, I think we can all agree, a sensible plan.'

Sensible for sure. Weight problems are a significant issue for many people and the risks that come with being morbidly obese can be extremely serious. In my experience it can sometimes be the symptom of more complex mental health problems. Self-harming doesn't just come in the form of cutting open your forearms. Food can be a great comforter – indeed, ingesting some high-fat, high-calorie foods can result in the body releasing endorphins and other 'feel-good' chemicals. Some nutrition scientists even use the phrase 'ingestion analgesia', literally pain relief from eating, to describe that blissed out 'food coma' that we all experience from time to time. I have known a number of patients who used eating as a crutch, in just the same way as they might alcohol or drugs, and it was nigh-on impossible to combat the eating without first addressing the state of mind that led to it.

'Have you always had problems with your weight?' I asked.

'No. In my youth I was slim and fit and beautiful and could climb mountains. Now I have become one.' He laughed, and it was such a huge and joyous sound it was impossible not to smile in response. Some people are blessed with infectious humour and Mr Khan was certainly one of them. But again, I knew well enough that that itself could be a sign of some problem deeper inside. There are those who are simply jolly however, and I hoped he was one of them.

His face became slightly more serious. 'I grew up in Pakistan, in the north, amongst the Hindu Kush. Do you know of them?'

'No,' I admitted. 'Sorry.'

'Mountains,' he continued, 'beautiful but dangerous. Which is how they get their name, it means: "Hindu Killer". Fancy! What sort of name is that for a place? Would you live in a nice little town called Doctor Slaughter? No. You are too sensible. But that is where I was born and I was young and I was beautiful and I was thin.' He leaned forward and whispered. 'It did not last. My family moved to Karachi and there I discovered good food. Wonderful food. The best in the world. Have you eaten in Karachi?'

'No.'

'Of course not, look at you! You cannot have been to Karachi! If you had been to Karachi, you would not be so slim. Karachi has all the best restaurants. Except maybe for London. I moved to London fifteen years ago, you see, and discovered cream tea. Do you like cream tea?'

'Yes,' I admitted. 'I love cream tea .'

'I love it too!' He exclaimed. 'Take a cake, decide it is not being all it can be. Spread jam on it. And still, it could be more! Lazy cake! Bad cake! Cake? Pull up your breeches and your socks! Add cream! Clotted no less, like my arteries! Ah …' His face became dreamy. 'One day I will revolutionise the world and discover how it is then possible to deep-fry it. But, until then, the scone is complete. Yes, cream tea. It's very funny.' He sighed. 'Well, not so funny perhaps. Not now. But there, life is full of regrets. Cream tea and selling cocaine. These are my biggest regrets.'

Mr Khan certainly loved to talk.

'You sold drugs?'

'I did. You must hate me. I hate me, it is a stupid thing, a horrible thing, but there we are. Life is full of wrong things. I was caught, sentenced, and spent five years in Wormwood Scrubs before being transferred here.'

'Oh, I've been working in the Scrubs for the past few years,' I told him. 'And still work there three days a week.'

'Ah! Then you know it!'

'I do, and I'm surprised our paths haven't crossed before.'

'I was busy,' he said, and his face fell. 'Eating. And while the snake-filled forest may be in London ... ' He leaned forward. 'That it is where the name comes from, did you know? Wormwood? *Snake* wood, hundreds of years ago! But yes, while it may be in the finest city for food there is, it is not, itself, a good place to eat. No. It is a very bad place to eat if you need to lose weight. Some of the food actually tasted good, but that is only the fried food and carbohydrates. I also bought a lot of food from the canteen, especially Pot Noodles. I think I became addicted to them. A kettle and a spoon and I was in nirvana. Too many biscuits and loads of chocolate as well,' he admitted.

I glanced at the clock, terribly aware that I'd started enjoying myself, listening to him, and the allotted time for his appointment was rapidly running out.

'At least I never resorted to catching pigeons through

the window!' he announced at some volume. 'Killing them and then boiling them in my kettle, like some prisoners did. I could never do that,' he said, looking disgusted.

'Oh, that's dreadful,' I replied, revolted by the thought. 'I'd heard of such a thing going on, but couldn't bear to believe it was true.'

'Yes, sadly it went on,' he replied, nodding. 'Quite horrible!'

He sighed, deflated at the thought of boiled birds. 'So, as you can see, I am now paying the price for my excesses. But I am delighted to say that I have been on a diet for the past two weeks, since I saw the dietician, and already feel better. She was really encouraging, and I feel very positive now and motivated to get fit!' He punched the air, his confidence returned.

I clicked on his notes to find the entry from Rowena, the dietician who worked at Huntercombe two mornings a week.

'It's a new start,' he continued. 'A new me. Soon I will be beautiful and thin again. *Soon*,' he said with a big smile.

'Well,' I told him, 'I think it's wonderful that you seem so positive and motivated to change your life. It really will be worth it and you will feel so good. I am sure you are aware of all the health risks associated with being overweight, aren't you?'

'Yes, Doctor, most learned, kind woman, I am,' he replied, voice sombre. 'I have done a lot of reading and Rowena gave me quite the terrifying lecture as well. She is kind, yes, but also very terrifying on the bitter and miserable subject of arteries.' His fingers tapped on his thighs. 'She also arranged for me to have my bloods checked to make sure that I have not done too much damage to myself. Such an enthusiastic gourmand of all, was I. But apparently no damage done, which is a relief and a small miracle, I think. It just goes to show, it's never too late to change!'

'Certainly isn't, Mr Khan, certainly isn't.' I glanced at the clock. His appointment had now run out. 'So, how can I help you today?'

'Oh yes!' He held his hands up to his face in a wonderfully theatrical gesture of shock. 'I should stop wasting your time and get to the point. I do love to talk, I'm afraid. Love it almost as much as food. So ...' He leaned forward again, his voice dropping. 'What's bothering me badly is a terrible rash at the top of my legs which is really sore and itchy. It's been there for ages and I just can't seem get rid of it. I've applied more cream to my legs than I have to scones, which, I can assure you, is a very worrying sign.'

'Would you like to show me?' I asked.

For a moment Habib looked worried, and I spotted the first clear chink in his happy armour. For all his bravado he was clearly slightly embarrassed to let me examine him.

'I suppose that would be sensible,' he said, but still he hesitated.

'Would you like a chaperone?' I asked.

He laughed. 'No thank you. Dear me, no. Let's not

start selling tickets. The fewer people that have to bear the business the better, I think.'

He stood up with sudden determination and pulled down his oversized tracksuit bottoms to reveal an extensive rash on the upper, inner aspect of his thighs. It extended to the large fold of abdominal skin overhanging his groin area, which, with a further twinge of embarrassment, he lifted up to show me.

As he did so an awful smell escaped into the room. The skin beneath was bright red and moist, with some raw areas that were oozing a little blood. It looked so sore, and I suspected that the rash was likely to have been there for some considerable time.

'It's serious, isn't it?' he asked, struggling to hold up the excess flesh. 'I knew it must be. To begin with it wasn't so bad, but I scratched at it and it worsened and worsened, and then I became worried that it may be cancer, because it looks so terrible, so raw, and the smell! And I grew frightened.' The garrulous Habib was gone now, to be replaced by someone just as talkative but filled with fear rather than joy. 'I was terrified at the thought of show-ing a doctor because I was too scared! It's always better to know the truth, that's what people say. Idiots! Fools! Who wants to hear that sort of truth? So, I waited and waited and—'

'It's not cancer, Mr Khan,' I said, interrupting. 'In fact, it's a very common rash called intertrigo that usually affects areas of the body where the skin rubs together and traps moisture. It is also relatively easy to treat.' I tried to make my voice as gentle, as reassuring as possible. 'So, you can stop worrying.'

I thought he was going to burst into tears he looked so relieved.

'Really?' he asked. 'Most learned and kindly doctor, is that really true?'

'It's true,' I said. 'So pull up your trousers and pants.'

'Oh!' It suddenly occurred to him that he should do just that. 'That's the best news I've heard in a long time,' he announced as he tucked himself back in and sat down.

He was actually quiet as I explained the treatment and how to try to prevent it recurring. Slightly in shock, I think the terrible fear that it was cancer that he had held onto for so long – most likely many months – had been taken away to be replaced by something so simple and unimportant.

'You are a marvel,' he said. 'Better than all the cream teas in the Cotswolds.'

'I'll see you again in a few weeks to review the rash and the rest of your blood results,' I said. 'As there a couple that are not back yet. Hopefully when I see you again you will have lost some more weight too?'

'You can be sure of it, Doctor Brown!' he said, getting to his feet. 'I may even be able to fit into your normal chair!'

He stepped outside and then, immediately, his head reappeared. 'But probably not, so it might be worth borrowing that one again? Maybe?'

'I'll always make sure you can sit with me, Mr Khan,' I reassured him. 'See you in a few weeks.'

After completing my notes on Mr Kahn, I returned the chair to admin and proceeded to work my way through the rest of the morning's patients. I had only seen one patient so far and was already massively behind. If I wanted to keep my appointment with David at lunchtime I needed to try to get back on track.

Fortunately, the rest of the morning was relatively straightforward and as the clock approached half past twelve, I heaved a sigh of relief that I had no more patients to see.

I logged out of the computer and dashed over towards David's office, hoping that nothing had got in the way of his schedule and that he was still able to chat.

'Doctor!' he called, standing in the doorway, as I approached his office. 'You'll be pleased to hear that Mr Grace was admitted into hospital without a hitch and that his tests are ongoing.'

'Ah! Good,' I said. 'Glad to hear it. I'm sure they'll get to the bottom of it.'

'Sure to,' he agreed, stepping back to let me into his office.

'Take a seat, ,' he said gesturing to the spare chair.

I sat down, as did he.

'Now,' he said, pulling over a small Tupperware box, 'you'll forgive me if I eat my lunch, but I'm not going to have time otherwise. There's been a fuss over the deportation of one of the men, and my lunch break is bound to be cut short by someone from the Home Office wanting me to sort it.'

'Are you sure it's convenient to talk?' I asked. 'I don't want to add to your worries.'

'You're not,' he insisted, popping the lid off his lunchbox. 'You're distracting me from them. You wanted to talk about Mr Aboah?'

'I can't stop thinking about him,' I admitted. 'His cancer is so advanced, and he is running out of time. Is there any way of him being released early on compassionate grounds? Let him go back to Ghana so that he can die surrounded by his family, not here in the UK? He doesn't have much time left to serve, anyway.' I realised I had barely paused for breath.

David took a bite of his rice cake. Chewed it. Swallowed. Then he placed the rice cake back in the Tupperware box and closed the lid.

'Back at the Scrubs,' he said, 'when you wanted to send the prisoner to hospital...'

'Yes?' I was worried what he might say. Had he actually been livid about that all this time? Was he about to drag it back up and berate me for it?

'I think,' he continued, 'that I must have seemed as if I had no compassion whatsoever.'

'Oh no!' I said. 'Not at all!'

'And yet, you were worried this morning that I was going to be angry again, weren't you?'

'Maybe a little,' I admitted.

'And this business with Mr Aboah,' he said. 'You half expect me to just dismiss it, don't you?'

I sighed. 'Yes, I suppose. But that's not because of any perception of you.'

I shouldn't be here.

How often did I feel concerned to push my thoughts? My beliefs? It wouldn't stop me. I couldn't let it stop me; there were usually people's lives at stake. But yes, how often did it feel almost impossible? Feel as if I was causing a problem. As if I were speaking out of turn.

'I'm aware I'm probably overstepping my mark,' I said.

'By caring for one of your patients?' David said. 'Rubbish. You're no more overstepping your mark as Prison Doctor than I am as Governor. Mr Aboah needs help. You can probably guess how difficult and how complicated the process will be. But we have to try. Of course, we do.'

I wanted to hug him ...

'Oh, that's wonderful! Thank you so much. Is there anything you need from me?'

David stared sadly at his lunchbox. 'Not unless you have a spare baguette.'

Unfortunately, the spring in my step that I had in the knowledge that something definite was happening for Kofi Aboah, didn't last long, as the afternoon surgery was a nightmare.

With patient after patient, I began to fall behind schedule. Then, halfway through the clinic, I clicked on the appointments ledger and saw that the next patient on the list was a young Malaysian man called Chan Keen, who according to the ledger, spoke no English.

Carrying out a consultation via an interpreter usually meant that it took at least twice as long. My heart sank.

I went to the door to call his name, 'Mr Keen?' I asked.

A man stood up and started walking towards me.

'Please come in and take a seat, I won't be long,' I said, indicating for him to sit down, hoping that he might perhaps understand just a little English. He looked back at me with a blank expression.

He was of small stature, very slight in build, and his clothes looked far too big for him.

I smiled at him, hoping to make him feel a little less scared while I pulled the phone a bit closer so that I could dial the translation service. It was one of those splayed 'spider' phones that tend to be used for conference calls, a big speaker at the heart of it, which was so much better than having to pass a handset from one person to another.

I dialled the number and we sat and waited for some time for it to answer. All I could do while we waited was smile at him until I began to feel a bit stupid. I decided to stare at my feet instead. Then the wall. Then my feet again. All the while, both of us sat awkwardly together listening to the ring tone.

Finally, a voice at the other end answered.

'Hello,' came the voice, a particularly tired and jaded sounding woman. 'You're through to Vox translate, please can I have your name, location and reference number?'

Without this it was not possible to use the service, so I rattled off the necessary information, feeling a little like a prisoner of war, reciting name rank and serial number.

'Thank you, Dr Brown,' said the voice, my credentials having been checked. 'And what language do you require?'

If nothing else, the long wait meant that I'd had more than enough time to check the patient's notes. There are many living languages in Malaysia, after all.

'Southern Min, please.'

'No problem. Please hold the line.'

There was a click, and then Mr Keen and I were treated to a rather crackly instrumental version of the love theme from the movie *Titanic*. 'My Heart Will Go On' ... and on ... and on ...

While we waited, I glanced again at his notes on the computer. He hadn't been at Huntercombe long, having only recently transferred from HMP Pentonville.

When he had first arrived in custody there had been concern because he had expressed suicidal thoughts, so much so in fact that, for a while, he was even on a constant watch.

He was serving a sentence for trying to buy Duty Free items using a fraudulent credit card. It seemed such an absurd crime, somehow – such a pitiful way of throwing away his freedom. I thought of the shops in the airport, places to kill time and empty wallets while you waited. What did I normally buy when travelling abroad? Maybe a cheap bottle of some spirit or other, maybe some perfume. Nothing I would want to be locked up for, certainly.

He shuffled in his seat and appeared to be in some discomfort.

The most striking thing about him was an obvious swelling of his thyroid gland.

His eyes were also a bit protuberant and he was sweating slightly. I realised that the diagnosis was almost certainly staring right back at me.

Frustrated that we were still waiting for a translator to be found, I decided to try passing the time by miming, which I found from past experience could come in quite useful.

First I tapped fast on my heart indicating a rapid heart rate. He nodded and tapped fast on his heart too.

He then clutched his abdomen and leaned forward in pain.

I mimed vomiting but he shook his head.

Then, to my surprise, he sat on his hands and made a loud raspberry sound, miming what I presumed was diarrhoea.

Just as he did that, the music stopped and a voice at the other end of the phone said, 'Hello, I am your South Min interpreter. How can I help you today?'

'Hello!' I said, possibly slightly too enthusiastically, unsure of how much of Mr Keen's bowel discomfort the translator was already aware of. 'My name is Doctor Brown and I have Mr Keen with me.'

'Can you please ask him how I can help him today?'

'Of course,' the translator replied,

After a few minutes I was told that Mr Keen was worried that he had lost a lot of weight and had diarrhoea.

I then began to run through the questions I needed to ask and, between the three of us, the answers started flowing and at last we were able to get somewhere. As was so often the case, the ten minutes allocated for the appointment had long since run out, but at least I was able to confirm my suspicions: Mr Keen had an overactive thyroid, which had already been diagnosed back in Malaysia, but he hadn't told anyone about it since arriving in the UK. He had been without his medication for at least six months and was in a bad way as a result.

In addition to how bad he was, physically, like so many of the people I try to help he was in a much worse way mentally. Once he had begun speaking to the translator, he was finding it hard to stop. To suddenly be in a position where he could speak his own language, pour out his thoughts and fears. Panicked sentence after panicked sentence flowed out of him, so much so that I think the translator must have been struggling to keep up.

'What's he saying?' I asked eventually as I needed to know how to steer the conversation on to the right path.

'It's to do with his mother,' the translator replied. 'He's really worried about her back home in Malaysia. She's very ill and, without him there, she has nobody to look after her.

'Well, hopefully he'll be returning soon and will be able to care for her,' I said, hoping it was true, although it wasn't clear from his notes exactly how much longer he had to serve.

'He's terrified about that, too,' the translator continued, 'as apparently he owes money. A lot of money. Once he's back home, there are a lot of people who are going to want to see him. I get the impression that he fears they will kill him. He says that he committed the crime because he was desperate to get out of debt, but now he's in even worse trouble.'

'Oh, that's shocking! I am so sorry to hear that,' I said, once again coming up against a problem that I couldn't possibly solve. 'Can you tell him I will ask someone from the mental health team to come and see him?'

She communicated this to Mr Keen.

'He says thank you,' she told me. 'And also muttered something about that being unlikely to help him, unless the mental health team had twenty thousand Malaysian ringgits they can lend him.'

'It's the best I can do,' I told her.

'Of course, it is,' she replied. 'Don't worry, I think he's just … he's very anxious.'

'I know,' I continued. 'Can you please also explain to him that it is very important that he gets back on the medication to control his overactive thyroid? I will prescribe tablets for him which will control all the symptoms he is suffering from and, on that, he will soon feel much better. But please, emphasise to him how important it is to take the medication every day – he can't just stop taking it.'

'I'll tell him,' the translator said, proceeding to talk to Mr Keen, who nodded and waved his hand as if it was the very least of his concerns.

'Can you also let him know that I will arrange for him to have blood tests done tomorrow,' I asked.

'Sure, of course.' She broke off to update him and he smiled back nervously at me in acknowledgement before giving a reply to the translator.

'He says he is very grateful and to thank you for your help.'

I smiled back at him, continuing to explain to the interpreter that he would need regular blood tests to monitor the treatment, and that I would refer him to a nearby hospital to see a specialist.

When, eventually, I felt we had covered all the facts and established a plan for his care I thanked the interpreter and finally ended the call.

Mr Keen looked so sad as he nodded to me with a faint smile and made his way back towards the door and the waiting room outside. He looked so small and timid, arms folded, shoulders hunched, as if trying not to take up too much space in the room. My heart felt so heavy at the thought of how bleak his future must seem to him, and as he walked away I felt that all too familiar feeling that I was powerless to really help him.

The rest of the afternoon was a case of trying to catch up. I hate being late and was conscious that people were outside waiting, possibly getting angry and impatient that I was running so late. Still, medicine can't be rushed, especially when some of it has to be conducted in mime.

I had reason to use the translation service another three times during the clinic, as I needed help from Romanian, Lithuanian and Vietnamese interpreters. The day just felt like it was getting worse and worse when, after waiting on the phone for about five minutes, I was told that a Vietnamese interpreter was not available, and that I would have to try again later. There was simply no time for that, so I had little choice but to rely once more on my miming skills which, by then, were beginning to become quite impressive, I have to admit.

By the time I had finished seeing the last patient of the day, I felt totally exhausted and drained of all emotion.

I had heard so many different stories, and of so many different struggles. The worst thing, however, was that I had felt time and time again that I had so little to offer most of the people I had seen that day, because their underlying problem was way beyond the assistance of medicine.

Working at Huntercombe really did come with a different set of challenges, and I felt so tired and wondered if – well, feared really – that perhaps I wasn't able to cope with it mentally and emotionally.

Their stories were so affecting, and I was frustrated that I couldn't do more, afraid that I was failing these men. Maybe I just wasn't tough enough for it.

But then, heading back to my car, the thought of Kofi Aboah dropped into my head. I had to persevere a bit longer. I didn't want to abandon him and the thought of trying to reunite him with his family gave me a reason to carry on.

At least for a while.

Chapter Five

'Dr Brown!' called a voice across the courtyard. A flurry of pigeons took to the air in panic and, for one nauseous moment, I was reminded of my conversation with Habib Khan, and I felt I could almost smell the bubbling, foul aroma of kettle-boiled birds.

I looked towards the voice and was pleased to see Daniel Kobe, hands thrust in his tracksuit pockets, huge grin on his face. Had a prisoner ever looked so at ease, so happy to be right where he was? By sharp contrast, next to him was Kofi. And while he was also smiling, the good humour was forced. The swelling on his neck was even more pronounced and his skin had a pallid, grey look to it.

I walked over. 'Hello, you two, you've met then?'

'Of course, a little corner of Ghanaian sunshine in this gloomy, gloomy place,' said Daniel, gesturing around at the grey, wintry courtyard. 'We shine bright enough even to wake this place up a little, huh?'

'You certainly do,' I agreed. I turned to Kofi. 'And how are you feeling, Mr Aboah?'

'The new pills are much better, thank you, Doctor Brown. The pain is easier to bear now.'

It was such a relief to hear that I had, at least, managed to ease his pain, even if only a little. When the one thing to offer someone is the ability to cope, any small success is welcome.

'Just doing my job,' I assured him. 'But I'm really pleased to hear that the pain is a bit more manageable now.'

He shook his head. 'A little more than just doing your job, I think.'

Daniel nodded. 'She is a good doctor, my friend, maybe she has a bit of sunshine too, eh?'

'You charmer, Mr Kobe,' I said, feeling a little embarrassed. 'What are you both up to today?'

'I am going to introduce Kofi to his new best friend.'

'Really?' I replied. 'And who's that?'

Daniel smiled. 'Mr Kuti.'

'That's nice,' I said, not having the first idea who Mr Kuti might be. 'You can never have enough friends.'

While I was ignorant of the man in question, Kofi clearly wasn't. 'You didn't tell me it was Mr Kuti!' he replied, shocked. 'Such an important man? I can't believe I am actually going to meet him. It will be such a great honour.'

'No,' Daniel shrugged, as if this were all just the sweetest and simplest thing. 'It was going to be a surprise, but now you know!'

For a moment I felt awkward, embarrassed even, that I didn't know who this Mr Kuti was. Clearly, I was missing something.

'He is a very powerful man, Doctor Brown,' said Daniel, clearly registering my confusion. '*Very* powerful. One of the most important people in Ghana. If anyone can help Kofi, it is him.'

'Well, that all sounds wonderful.' I still didn't really know what to say. 'And where is Mr Kuti?'

'He is in the cell along the corridor from mine,' said Daniel.

'He's a prisoner?' I asked, unable to quite keep the surprise from my voice.

'Yes,' Daniel replied with a big smile, as if this fact made it all the better.

'But that must be a mistake' Kofi said, his face so serious, so earnest. 'He's far too important to be in prison.'

Daniel wasn't quite so sure of that, I could tell; there was a look in his eyes that suggested he knew only too well that Mr Kuti had earned his place in a Huntercombe cell. 'A business matter,' he said, feigning dismissal. 'These things can happen. Complications. Misunderstandings. An error in the counting. But it is of no matter; Mr Kuti has not let it hold him back. He is as important as he ever was.'

'Well, we mustn't be late for him,' said Kofi, clearly very excited at the thought of who he was about to meet.

Daniel smiled. 'It is not a long walk, my friend, nowhere is in here!' He laughed and they moved off across the courtyard, Daniel calling back over his shoulder, 'See you soon, Doctor Brown!'

I watched them go for a moment, then continued on my way towards Healthcare.

Passing the library, I noticed Asma standing outside. She was shaking a paperback book violently in one hand, as if trying to remove dust from it.

'Morning!' I called.

'Souvenirs!' she shouted back, holding up the book. 'You wouldn't believe what ends up inside some novels by the time they're returned.'

I veered closer; I had a few minutes to spare.

'I'm not sure I want to know,' I said, dreading to think what she might be referring to.

'Oh,' she replied, 'don't worry, nothing *biological*. Nothing that might need burning. Those sections get torn out and kept, I certainly never see them again. Some writers lose more weight than others. I had to throw away a Jean M. Auel the other day that had shed a couple of hundred pages during its time on the stacks. Lots of cave girl action in a Jean M. Auel.'

'I haven't read any,' I admitted.

'It's all bear skins and bare bums,' she said. 'You're not missing much. But this' – she held up the book and I could see it was a 'searing true-life account of life in Columbia's drug cartels' – 'is not that sort of book. This is the sort of book that people like to send us because it's full of criminals feeling terribly sorry for themselves and wishing they had never set foot on the path to iniquity. It also features lots of guns and walloping great sacks of cocaine.'

'Oh.' Definitely not my type of book.

'Yes, and in this *precise* edition, this extremely limited edition of one, is some form of yeasty residue that, I am fairly sure, is dry flavouring from a Pot Noodle.' She sniffed the book. 'Yes, definitely. Bombay Bad Boy.'

'I'm sorry?'

'The flavour, Doctor Brown, the flavour. Am I to understand you're not a connoisseur of the dehydrated noodle snack?'

'Not anymore. I used to eat them when I worked in hospital as a junior doctor a very long time ago. Back in those days I don't think I ever ate a proper meal. I just grabbed whatever I could, whenever I could,' I said, briefly reliving the memories of my early days in medicine. Bowls of cereal and toast were two other favourites.

'Well, you just ask anyone in here, they'll tell you. You don't know what you're missing!' she said, laughing. 'Anyway, how are you enjoying it here?'

'Fine, I think,' I said. 'Just trying to do my bit.'

'It gets to you though, doesn't it?' she said. 'This place. It's not like the other prisons I've worked in. The atmosphere, the … I don't know … all these little microcosms of countries, all with their own problems, their own identities.' She waved the book in the air again, this time as if trying to knock her own thoughts away, as if they were flies. 'I mean … don't get me wrong, prisons are *always* like that,' she continued. 'There are always groups. Humans like to clump together, don't they? It makes them feel safer. Stronger. Of course, that's going to happen in a place like this. Still, it's definitely *different* here somehow. There's more of them, of course. So many different communities, so many different countries. Did you ever see that old TV show, *The Prisoner*? It reminds me of that, sometimes, this whole world of a population, all bundled together into one tiny space. Even then,' she continued, still not settling on a thought, 'I don't think it's that. It's not just about where these people are from. What is it?' And finally, I sensed she actually did want my thoughts on the matter. 'What is it that makes this place so different?'

'Perhaps it's because most people here are getting towards the end of their sentence?' I suggested. 'At least they should be. This isn't like most prisons, where there are lots of people who have years and years left to serve. That must change how people act and behave to a certain extent, don't you think?'

'Definitely,' Asma agreed, nodding and thinking. 'That probably has got a lot to do with it.'

'And so many of them don't want to leave at all,' I added. 'Well, they don't want to leave in the way they *have* to. They don't want to go back to the countries they're being sent to. That certainly seems to add a very heavy level of stress to a lot of the people I become involved with.'

'Sure, sure,' Asma agreed, 'but there are also a lot that *do* want to get back to their home country, you know there's nothing so useful as consistency in this place. Maybe that's it, maybe that's the salt and vinegar on the chips of this place.' She sighed. 'Oh well, enough of this hanging about, I have to get on and clean the Grishams. Far too thick a Grisham, you can squish a lot of rubbish into one, like foul-smelling pressed junk flowers. See you around.' She headed back inside and, with a smile, I continued on towards Healthcare.

I stepped through the entrance and locked the gate and then the door behind me. I came face to face with Rosemary. There were many people who found her very intimidating and who might even experience mild panic to come face to face with her. She had that effect on people because of her very strong personality, especially if she had taken against someone. To suddenly find yourself in her gaze was rather like being on the end of an antiseptic-smelling hard stare.

Luckily for me, I had never found myself on the wrong side of her, thank heaven.

'Hello, you,' she said. 'I was waiting for you to come in. We've got news about the patient you sent to hospital the other day.'

'Oh?' I thought back to poor Akeem Grace, and how very unwell he was.

Had he had appendicitis after all?

'He started coughing up blood almost as soon as he got there, apparently,' she explained.

'Definitely not appendicitis, then,' I said, only too well aware of the many times that what appeared to be appendicitis would prove not to be the case after all. Rosemary shook her head. 'No. After all the usual investigations it turned out that he had haemophilus influenzae pneumonia, complicated by sepsis.'

Haemophilus influenzae type B used to be a serious problem in the UK, particularly in children. The bacteria could lead to a number of different conditions (pneumonia and blood poisoning in Akeem's case). In 1992 it became part of the routine immunisations for babies which, thankfully, means such infections are now rare for people born in the UK.

'Which would account for why he was obviously so ill,' I said. 'Thank goodness he got to hospital in time.'

'Saved his life, I reckon,' she said. 'A good morning's work before you'd even started your surgery.' She grinned. 'Keep it up!'

The surge of relief that washed over me, knowing he was okay, was huge. It doesn't matter how long I do this job, nor how many patients I see, there is always the biggest, all-consuming relief when I know that a decision I made was the right one. The thought of what might have happened if he hadn't gone to hospital didn't bear thinking about.

'Well at least the boss will know that it was the right decision to send him in,' I said, always thankful for not wasting everyone's time. It was hard to forget the difficult decisions and conversations I had been involved with over the years, regarding prisoners being sent to hospital. On a couple of occasions, I had even ended up in tears.

I shouldn't be here.

'He certainly does,' a distinctive voice said behind me. Not only were those shoes shiny, but they were also stealthy.

'Hi, David,' I said. 'How are you? Don't often see you in Healthcare this early in the day.'

He smiled. 'No, who needs a governor underfoot?'

'Quite,' said Rosemary with a big, dangerous grin.

David was not someone affected by the presence of Rosemary. He just smiled at her then turned back to me. 'I was hoping that you might have a few spare minutes for a quick chat?'

'Of course,' I said. 'I was just going to my room to log on. Is it okay to chat there?'

'Perfect.' He turned slightly towards Rosemary. 'Nurse Walbrook, a pleasure as always.'

'Likewise, Governor,' she said, that fixed grin still in place. Rosemary was never quite sure about governors; they controlled budgets, they made decisions, most of all they might not always agree with the decisions *you* made. That was all reason enough as far as Rosemary was concerned to keep on the back foot.

We walked along the corridor and I unlocked my room, gesturing for David to go in. He sat down in the blue chair next to the desk. It seemed odd to see him sitting where the patients sat, and I felt like asking him if he had any medical issues, but resisted the temptation.

'So what's new?' I asked. 'Any problem?' I suddenly

realised I was extremely nervous, worried about what he might have to tell me.

'No problem at all,' he replied, reassuringly. 'I just wanted to talk to you about Mr Aboah.'

'I just saw him in the courtyard,' I explained, 'with Daniel Kobe.'

'Ah yes.' David nodded. 'Nice man. The officer on his wing tells me that Mr Kobe has been looking out for Mr Aboah. He seems to be coping a bit better now, integrating more.'

That was definitely nice to hear. 'It was good to see him look a little happier this morning,' I agreed.

It occurred to me that David was exactly the man to shine a little light on the conversation I'd had with Daniel and Kofi.

'Actually,' I said, 'can I ask you something? Mr Kobe was talking about introducing Kofi to someone on the same wing, a Mr Kuti? They both seemed very impressed by him, as if he was someone really important.'

David nodded. 'Our Mr Kuti is something of a VIP in the prison. Works with the government in Ghana and is worth a fortune. Got fingers in all sorts of pies.'

'It must be a real shock for him to be in prison then.'

'Oh, I don't know about that, he's as crooked as they come! The real surprise is that he got caught doing it! And caught over here for that matter. Counterfeit money of all things, as if he hadn't enough of the real thing.'

'The stories I hear about people's lives will never cease

to amaze me,' I said. 'However old I am, I always hear something new to surprise me. No wonder they are so fascinated by him!'

'Yes, all the Ghanaian prisoners here treat him like royalty, unfortunately. We discourage it as best we can, but it's hard to control really. They clean his cell for him, buy him treats from the canteen, make sure he gets a large portion from the servery at meal times. All trying to find favour, no doubt. You know what it's like, as far as most of them are concerned this is someone who has the money to completely change their lives; they'll do almost anything for a chance at that.'

'Understandable. I hope he doesn't plan on taking advantage of Mr Aboah, though.'

'I wouldn't have thought so. Mr Kuti is quite a nice man, actually. Besides, he doesn't need anything from him. He's not got long before we return him to Ghana, and he'd certainly be in a position to help Mr Aboah's family as and when he does.' David couldn't keep the sadness from his face. 'Even if Mr Aboah doesn't manage to eventually join him.'

'Really?' I asked. 'It's not going well then?'

This was the last thing I wanted to hear. Had I assumed that the simplicity, the basic necessity, the *humanity* of this case would see everything, and everyone, swing into place to allow Kofi Aboah to see his family again before he died?

'I've been working hard on it,' David said. 'Because I feel as strongly as you do that it's the right thing to do. I won't give up without a fight, you can be assured of that.'

'That is so good to know,' I told him. 'Not that I ever doubted it.'

'Your faith in me is flattering.' He sighed and leaned back in his chair. 'I understand the legal difficulty,' he continued. 'Of course, I do. We are trying to make something rather complicated and extreme happen.'

'Early release?' I said. 'Surely there are all sorts of mitigating factors for that? Good behaviour for one.'

'But we're not talking about a time frame within the usual legal parameters of release,' David explained. 'We're asking for him to be released *much* earlier than that. We're effectively asking for his sentence to be drastically altered.'

'But surely,' I argued, 'in these circumstances it hardly matters? Mr Aboah is going to be dead long before his release date, so the normal rules can't really apply,' I said, hoping it were true.

'Well, that's the point, isn't it? The 'normal rules' as you say are points of law and the Home Office doesn't make a habit of breaking the law! However logical it is to have him released early, however considerate and humane, we can't simply ignore the law to do so. I'm working on finding a precedent but, so far, no luck.'

'So what can we do?' I asked.

'He would certainly be eligible for the Early Release Scheme.'

'Which is?'

'A scheme specifically for foreign national prisoners. It allows those awaiting deportation to leave much earlier than their release date.'

'How early?'

'Up to a maximum of two hundred and seventy days before the midpoint of their sentence.'

'They would leave before their sentence was half served? There has to be a catch.' It seemed far too good to be true.

David smiled. 'Not a catch exactly but, yes, he has to fit a number of criteria. He has to have served at least a quarter of his sentence and not be serving a sentence for a breach of previous release terms. He's eligible but it does take time.'

'He hasn't got any!'

'I've already started the process. I'll have to speak to him, though, as it's vital he doesn't contest deportation – it's a voluntary scheme, so people who are contesting their return are not eligible.'

'Well, he's hardly likely to do that, is he? He wants to go home, that's the point.'

'I know.' David sighed. 'But I still need to go through it all with him. It's his decision to make, not mine. I can handle the paperwork, but he still has to want to apply. Though I'm sure he will.'

'Of course, he will.' I sighed. 'When you say it takes time, how long are we talking?'

David shrugged. 'Who can predict these things? There's a mountain of paperwork on the Home Office desk, we throw this on top of it and wait for it to work its way through.'

'You make it sound like digestion.' I smiled.

'Constipation, more like.' David returned my smile. 'I'll

also put him through for Facilitated Returns, a scheme that runs alongside the Early Release. Basically, it gives him a little bit of money to go back to. It's not a fortune – five hundred pounds on release and then a further thousand pounds after he's been in the country for a month. It all helps though.'

'Of course, it could make a major difference for his family.' I sat back in my chair. 'Let's hope he can keep going while we wait.'

'Once the paperwork is in motion I'll let you know,' he said. 'In the meantime, I'm trying to set up a video call for him to speak to his wife.'

'Video call? Wow, that would be wonderful for him. Imagine!'

'Frustrating,' he said, getting to his feet. 'It's proving an absolute nightmare to arrange their end.'

'Are they being difficult?'

'Well, not difficult so much as *complicated*. We need to schedule an appointment for his wife to go to the British embassy over there, the whole thing has to be done in very specific, very strict conditions. And each country has its own laws it needs to adhere to. Hopefully we'll get there, but right now they're not being terribly helpful.'

'Best of luck,' I said to him as he walked towards the door.

He opened the door and looked outside to a waiting room that was already filling up. 'I suspect it's you who'll need that, today,' he said with a smile. 'We'll catch up again soon.'

'Thanks, David,' I said, feeling so grateful that he was on my side, and clearly trying so hard to help. I looked around the waiting room; so many people who needed help. So much noise and so many new problems to hear about, but in that moment I could only think of one: Kofi Aboah. And we weren't even helping him to live. He was beyond that. All we could do, the very best we could do, was to help him to die well.

Chapter Six

'I don't want to die here.'

The woman speaking had skin as thin and soft as tissue paper. In fact, so delicate was it, so translucent, I could see the pulse in her wrist, that regular twitch, the reassuring tick and tock of life's clock. I watched it for a few moments:

Tick tock, tick tock, tick tock.

There was a brief sense of relief. The clock still running. Still counting out time.

Tick tock, tick tock, tick tock.

But, in truth, it had very few ticks left, and both she and I knew it.

All around us was the hustle and bustle of hospital life. There are few places as utterly lacking in silence as a hospital, often the very place where it is most needed. Even at night, the dramas of life and death bring the slap of rubber soles and the squeak and clatter of trolleys and beds. Vending machines clunk and whirr, drinks machines hiss and spit and froth. Strip lights buzz. Monitoring machines talk their language of beeps. Heavy doors grunt and sigh on hinges. Keyboards clatter typed data. Worse … these are halls of pain. There are sighs, cries, tears. People beg for relief. Muttered voices, wishing it would all change.

Hospitals are wonderful. Hospitals are amazing. Hospitals are hell.

'I know,' I told her. 'I shall do my very best to get you home.'

*

As a child, my grandmother lived with us for a number of years before she died at the age of eighty-nine. For the last few months of her life, I used to hear her in the night, a low, tired voice that she hoped would carry heavenward: 'Please, Jesus, take me this night.'

Eventually she got her wish, dying from pneumonia. I was twelve.

'Pneumonia,' my father said, 'is the old man's friend.'

He went on to explain that before antibiotics were discovered, it was regarded as a relatively quick and painless way to exit from this life, and that sometimes it was kinder to let nature take its course rather than to preserve life at all costs.

We spend most of our lives hoping to avoid death. Then, if we're unlucky, we learn better.

*

Two years after leaving my GP practice I became involved in a project that aimed to try and improve end of life care. Set up by Buckinghamshire Hospitals Trust, the project's main aim was to try and avoid hospital admissions if possible by developing safe and suitable alternative patient pathways, particularly for the elderly and vulnerable. A major part of the project was trying to enable people to be able to plan for their end of life care. If that's a conversation you think you never want to have, I can assure you the alternative can be worse.

My time was split between the community, care homes and hospitals and, frequently, once it came to the latter, the fight grew ever more difficult.

It was absolutely no fault of the staff, the doctors and nurses who did their very best to keep the oversubscribed hospitals functioning. It was just so hard for them to meet the demands they faced every day, with never enough beds for the number of patients needing them, let alone the crazy targets they had to achieve.

It was eye opening and deeply troubling to see frail, elderly, vulnerable, and often confused people at the end of their journey through life, lying on a trolley in a queue waiting to be assessed by the overstretched A & E team.

If they were then admitted to the ward some would remain there for weeks, often months, and during that time I would very often observe them deteriorate further, losing mobility and becoming more confused. They would end up far too frail to ever return home.

They were trapped in the system.

*

'Where do you want to be, Valerie?' I asked.

Valerie was staring at a poster on the wall, a woman with her head down, her hair hanging like a curtain over her face. 'Scared to go home?' the text on the poster asked.

'No,' Valerie whispered. I was confused for a moment and then, looking at the poster, realised I might understand.

'You'd rather be at home?' I asked her.

She nodded.

'*Bad Girls* is on,' she said, 'never miss *Bad Girls*. Filth.'

'Right.' I can't help but smile. 'Well, we'll have to see what we can do to get you back home.'

*

'Not long,' whispered Courtney, one of the community nurses. I nodded, glancing at the old man's son who was hunched over a boiling kettle in the corner of his father's kitchen. He'd been on the go now for thirty-six hours and desperately needed sleep. If Courtney was right he'd have the time he needed soon enough.

The son's name was Michael and he'd been expecting his father to die for two years.

I turned to look out of the kitchen window, a brief respite from the close atmosphere of the little two-up two-down. The smell of disappointing microwavable Thai curry lingered. Lemongrass, coriander and sweat.

I spotted a fox darting along the alley between this house and the one next door. Its fur was tousled and muddy. It was undernourished, desperately in need of a decently stocked binbag. It would get no joy here.

'When I was a kid all the placemats had fox hunting scenes on,' said Michael, having noticed the fox too. He poured water on three tea bags. 'You wouldn't get that now I don't think. Who'd want them? Couldn't move for them back then. Every country pub. Every crap café wanting to give its baked potato or omelette a look of class. Fox hunting. Red jackets and those... what do you call them, can't think of the word, posh trumpet...'

'Bugles,' I said.

'That's it. Like the crisps. Bugles.'

He just stared out of the window for a moment, steam from the three mugs in front of him rising up and diffusing in the light of the neon tube above us.

'I'm pretty sure,' he said eventually, 'that neither Mum nor Dad had been anywhere near a horse, let alone a fox. I mean... they grew up in Stepney. You don't get many horses in Stepney. What did they want with horses on the dinner table?'

He snapped out of it and began fishing for the teabags. He placed them neatly, gently, in a tiny saucer with the Crystal Palace football team logo on it.

'Is it okay?' he asked, oh so very quietly, 'to admit that I'm looking forward to it?'

'Your dad dying?' I asked.

He nodded. 'I say looking forward... you know what I mean... thinking it's good. For the best. I hate watching him have to go through this.'

'It is,' I agreed. 'Of course, it is. Your dad's been through so much.'

'Yes,' he nodded, staring down at the three teas, 'so much.'

He took a moment before speaking again.

'You never expect to see your dad in pain,' he said. 'Is that sexist? Maybe. Just gets hammered into you somehow. These last few months. Weakening. Suffering. I remember he...' emotion got in the way then for a moment and I could see his knuckles whiten against the cosmos of a mock black marble sideboard. 'When he had the colostomy bag fitted, he started showing it to me, explaining how it worked. Like I was a little kid again. Like I'd ever actually want to know. I decided then.' He sighed and went over to the fridge to fetch the milk. 'My dad should have died by now. The last two years has been a living hell for him'

'It's alright to want it to be over,' I said.

'I did the right thing then?' he asked. 'Stopping treatment?'

'You did what you thought he would want if he had been able to make that decision himself, but his dementia is far too advanced now. He's suffered enough. You acted with kindness. You acted with love.'

He nodded. 'I hope so. I knew it was right at the time. Absolutely knew it. The only decision to be made. But ever since, every single minute he's still alive, I wonder if I'm wrong. Is that normal? To be constantly thinking… what about now? If we started treatment again right *now* might it be in time? Might he carry on living?'

'That rather depends on how you define living. There has to be a quality of life. I would hate to be kept alive if I had no quality of life, Michael.'

'I had the same thing with my dog once,' he went on. 'I agreed with the vet to have him put down cos he had a tumour – cancer – but it seemed to take so long. Making him comfortable. Shaving his leg. Sedating him. Stroking him. It was excruciating… I'd made the decision, done what I thought was right and there he was. Still alive. Still breathing. Staring at me. And I can't know what he's thinking, I can't know if those eyes are asking me to save him. Because I still could, you know? I could change my mind. Because it's taking so long.

'I could change my mind. But I don't. Though I still think about it even though it's five years ago now. It haunts me. Right now. Now. For my dad…. There's still time. I could change my mind.'

Courtney came in. 'I think you should go upstairs, Michael.'

Michael stared at her, his face emptied while I was watching. Just hollowed out on the bone. 'I'm making tea,' he said, so quietly I almost couldn't hear him.

'I'll finish that,' I said, taking the teaspoon out of his hand and patting him softly on the arm. 'You go and see your dad.'

He walked slowly upstairs and I listened to his creaking footsteps all the way to the ceiling above me. Then I heard him sit down. That old chair of faded leather, that sighed with exhaustion every time someone landed on it.

Within five minutes the soft sound of his sobbing made its way through the ceiling.

*

'Please can I talk to someone about Valerie Walker,' I asked the receptionist. 'She came into A&E about an hour ago. I'm a GP working with the End of Life Project.'

'Right…' the receptionist sighed. 'Bear with me while I try and get her details up.'

'I know that she doesn't want to be admitted to hospital as she has made her wishes very clear to me,' I said. 'So, I need to try and get her home if possible.'

She tapped on the keyboard in front of her, eyes twitching as she scrolled quickly through the lists of information on the screen. 'You'll need to talk to whoever's dealing with her.'

'I know, and they're so busy it'll probably be hours,' I said, 'but if there's any way of speeding the process up I'd be so grateful.'

She nodded. 'I'll do my best.'

'That's really kind of you. Thank you so much.'

*

'I'm there now,' I told the doctor at the nursing home, turning off the car engine. 'I'll do my best.'

'I know you will,' he replied.

I hung up, unhooked the phone from the hands-free and put it in my bag. Climbing out of the car I dashed towards the hospital reception.

'I'm trying to find Adrian Leaman,' I told the receptionist. 'He's a resident at the White House nursing home. He is a ninety-one-year-old gentleman with dementia and was admitted after suffering from a dense stroke.'

'Got him,' said the receptionist. 'He's on Partridge Ward. Take the lift to the first floor, turn left and then keep going. You'll see Partridge on your right.'

'Thank you.'

The lift was, as is so often the way with a hospital lift, giving serious consideration to settling into a sulk. If you pressed each button twice it eventually considered paying attention to your request.

'Sorry about the beans,' said a young anaesthetist who had ridden up in the lift from the basement. She nodded at the rubber floor where a few baked beans sat looking awkward. She held up her polystyrene clamshell takeaway boxes. 'I sneezed, and the lid came off and some beans escaped!! Made a right mess.'

I nodded, not entirely sure what to say to that.

We arrived at the first floor and I stepped back to let an elderly woman with a large tartan handbag in.

'Sorry about the beans,' the anaesthetist was saying as I stepped out into the corridor and turned left.

The receptionist on Partridge Ward was doing her very best to finish a cheese salad sandwich. It sat in its cardboard triangle a foot away from the computer keyboard, one bite taken.

'I started that an hour ago,' she said as she looked up Mr Leaman. 'I don't even like cheese salad but it's all they had left. I'm determined to finish it now. Point of principle. He's in the first room on your right,' she pointed at the corridor behind me. 'Bed in the far left corner.'

I found Adrian Leaman, his eyes distantly staring at the corner of the room where a reflected light from another patient's watch kept dancing.

'Mr Leaman?' I asked, but there was no response.

'Doctor Brown?' a nurse asked as she entered the room. I nodded.

'Faroushka Sahid,' she said, shaking my hand. Her eyes were hooded, an extra-long, extra-difficult shift I was sure. I knew that look. 'You're with the project?' she asked, tactfully omitting its name.

'Yes, they called me from Mr Leaman's nursing home. There was some concern about getting hold of his family.'

'Have they managed?'

I shook my head. 'We're not actually convinced he has any.'

She sighed again. I suspected Faroushka often had cause to sigh.

'We're treating him for a chest infection,' she said, keeping her voice low. 'He's having IV antibiotics and we have inserted a PEG feeding tube as he is unable to swallow anything. We've also arranged a whole raft of investigations for him but, at the end of the day, we really need a family member to make a decision as to whether he would want us to actively treat him.'

'Because treating him's probably not the kindest thing to do,' I said. It wasn't a question; we were both only too aware of Mr Leaman's situation. He couldn't swallow, couldn't move his left side. Couldn't communicate in any way.

'But, until we're told otherwise, we're just going to have to keep going, of course.'

'Of course.'

She glanced at Mr Leaman, still staring at the corner of the room. 'God help him,' she said. 'It's not how I'd want to be spending the end of my days.'

'No,' I agreed. 'Who would?'

He died eight weeks later. Still in hospital. Alone.

'She'll be fine with us,' said Pete Walker, Valerie's son. 'I've spoken to the office and they're letting me work from home for a bit. Well, Mum's home, you know.'

I nodded. 'That's great.'

'My sister moved to Spain a couple of years ago but she's going to try and head over. It's not as easy for her work wise but, well, she's going to try.'

'Your mum will be so pleased,' I said, looking over his shoulder to Valerie who was slumbering in the passenger seat of Pete's car.

'Maybe,' he smiled. 'She always used to say we cluttered up the place. Whenever we visited. She basically lives for advocaat and telly.'

'*Bad Girls*,' I said.

He smiled. '*Bad Girls*, that's right. That and the racing and she's all set. Thanks for all your help.'

He opened the door of his car and clambered in.

'Come on lad,' Valerie said, stirring from her slumbers just before the door closed. 'We haven't time for you to be gallivanting and chatting up women. Time to get home and get curtains drawed.'

The door shut and I watched as they pulled away.

She passed away two months later. Happily.

I hope.

Working on the End of Life Project ranks as some of the most difficult and heart-breaking I've ever done but it was also some of the most fulfilling. I have always believed that helping someone to die well is such an important part of my job, not just for the patients but also their friends and families. Looking back now over my forty-one years in medicine, I regard it as some of the most rewarding work of my career.

Chapter Seven

HUNTERCOMBE
8 FEBRUARY 2014

I was feeling really hungry by the end of the morning clinic, so decided to pop over to the Rolls Inn to grab some lunch.

On the way, I saw Pastor Clive running along the corridor towards me, arms full of sheets of brightly coloured paper. His cheeks were puffed out and his wheezing travelled up the corridor towards me as if signalling the arrival of a train.

'Doc ... tor ... Brow ...' he huffed. 'Could I spea ...'

At which point he tripped on his own laces and went down in the middle of the corridor in a cloud of coloured paper, one last, jolly puff of smoke from his chimney stack.

I ran towards him, hoping that he hadn't hurt himself in the fall – he'd certainly gone down with some force.

'Careful, Pastor Clive,' I said as he tried to scrabble to his feet. 'Let me help you. Are you okay? I hope you haven't hurt yourself?'

'Oh, I'm fine, thank you,' he said, waving his hands in

the air. 'Nothing bruised but my ego, and that's an insult to God so it deserves a black eye from time to time.'

I started gathering his posters from the floor. 'Choir practice?' I asked.

'No, no, not today. That's Thursdays.' He started helping me gather the posters and passed them over so that he could tie his laces up.

I'd meant the posters, of course, but I saw now, as I picked up one that was facing the right way, that they were for something else entirely. 'SMILE DAY' it said in big red letters beneath the picture of a rising sun. There was then the date of a few weeks away, a row of smileys and, finally, 'WHAT DO YOU HAVE TO LOSE?' in matching red capitals.

'Smile day?' I asked.

'Yes!' he replied with a smile that proved he was, at least, an expert on the subject. 'Just something I'm trying. Too many frowns in the world at the moment. Far too many. It doesn't help, that's what I say. Frowns. Smiles are the way forward.'

'Well, yes,' I agreed. 'They're certainly much nicer to see about the place.'

'Aren't they?' he agreed.

'You wanted to talk to me?'

'Did I?' he was confused momentarily then his eyes snapped into focus. 'You're quite right! I did. About one of my flock, he's in a bad way.'

'Really? What's up with him?'

'Well...' As soon as he started talking I noted that he was gazing upwards and tapping his fingers together, an automatic process I assumed this overburdened man used to recall all the information he needed to the front of his brain so that he could repeat it. I wondered how many of his 'flock' were filed away in there, precious people all given their storage space and stories.

'I'm worried about him,' he said, 'because he's looking very gaunt and I'm sure he has lost a lot of weight, which is troubling because he was already very thin when I first met him. *Very* thin. He stoops. A lot of them do in here as I'm sure you know, they have few reasons to stand up straight. But Aaden stoops a *lot*. Properly hunched over. In the end I decided to ask him if he was feeling ill and he told me that his back is killing him and that he sweats so much at night he can't sleep.' For a moment his fingers tapped quicker. I imagined he was checking the brain's filing system for any last few pieces of important information. He found one.

'He also said that he feels really tired all the time,' he continued. 'But maybe that's because he's not been sleeping well. I do hope there is nothing seriously wrong with him. He's such a nice young man. Can you come and see him?'

'Well unfortunately I can't do "visits", as it were, because I don't have cell keys,' I explained. 'I'm really only permitted to see people in their cell if it is an emergency, or if they are too ill to come to Healthcare. Can he walk okay?'

'Yes, he can walk.' Pastor Clive started to rub at his hair. 'But I think he's too scared to make an appointment. Deep down I think he's frightened that there is something seriously wrong.' His face was such a picture of worry, a deep sadness furrowing every line. 'I hope to God that he hasn't got cancer,' he said, and for a moment or two he just kept rubbing his hair.

'He's originally from Somalia,' he continued, 'but he's been in the UK for a few years now, I think. I know he's getting worried about his deportation, so maybe that's what's wrong with him.' The worry was partially replaced by hope and, as if remembering his own posters, he began to smile. 'Better than a frown,' he said.

'Always,' I agreed. 'It certainly sounds as if he should come and see me. I can make him an appointment when I get back to my room, if you like?'

'That would be wonderful!' The smile widened.

'Okay,' I said, 'then let me write down his name, and also his prison number if you have it.'

'Thank you,' Pastor Clive said. 'I don't know his prison number, but his name is Aaden Waris Abdi.'

I took my biro out of my key pouch and, as I had no paper with me, jotted it down on the back of my hand.

'That's fine. I'm sure I will find him on the computer. Roughly how old is he?'

'Early twenties, and he's on Howard Wing if that helps?'

'Definitely.' I popped my pen back in my key pouch. 'Leave it with me, Pastor Clive.'

'Thank you. I'll tell him to expect an appointment and just hope he agrees to turn up.'

'I'm sure you'll manage to persuade him,' I said. His smile still in place, he nodded.

I handed him back his posters, which he hugged closely to his chest and carried on back down the corridor. I couldn't help noticing he had a slight limp following his fall.

'Remember!' he shouted back. 'Smile Day! What have you got to lose?'

He got one out of me then and there, I must admit. On the rare occasion that I saw him, he somehow always managed to make me feel happy. He seemed to radiate kindness and had such a cheerful and positive outlook on life.

When I arrived at the Rolls Inn, the queue had already spilled into the corridor. It was a really popular place for staff to eat, but also only a very small room, so it wasn't unusual to see a line of people snaking out of the door. I waited in the queue, trying to decide what to order. A ham and tomato sandwich for sure, but maybe I would treat myself to a slice of freshly baked cake too? As I reached the end of the queue, I saw that today's special was coffee and walnut that was looking positively gorgeous and impossible to resist ... But there were also doughnuts – another favourite. Oh dear, cake or a doughnut? Tough decision cake or a doughnut ...

'Doctor Brown!' someone shouted, and, dragging my thoughts away from the vital business of cake, I turned to see Habib Khan marching towards me, arms wide as if being reunited with an old friend he had known many years, as opposed to a doctor he'd consulted with only once. The thought of cake retreated to the back of my mind.

'Mr Khan,' I said, returning his enthusiasm, because it was all but impossible not to. 'How are you?'

'I'd show you,' he said, leaning forward to offer a stage whisper, 'but then I wouldn't want to excite the whole corridor.' He laughed uproariously and patted at the area on his legs where the rash had been. 'It has cleared up well,' he said. 'It is much improved.'

'Oh that's great, I'm so pleased,' I said.

'An absolute miracle! I was so sure it would be the death of me. But, no! A few weeks of your miracle unguent and I have the skin of a baby.' He shrugged. 'Well, a slightly scabby baby but it's getting there.' His face burst into even greater joy. 'And, even more importantly,' he continued, 'I have lost my first stone! How is that for news?'

'Excellent!' I told him. The queue was now much shorter and I realised I was going to have to order in a moment. I was torn. The cake looked really good but surely I should set a good example with my food choices, knowing how much Mr Khan would probably love to sink his teeth into a large slab of cake.

It was as if he'd read my mind. 'You are going to buy cakes?' he asked.

'Well,' I said, 'I'm probably just going to order a sand-wich.'

'Get a cake too,' he suggested. 'Take it from one who

knows. If you are able to eat one nice thing and still stay slim, you should. Enjoy the pleasures in life, Doctor, but don't let them rule you!' He laughed again and walked off, his laughter echoing all along the corridor.

It was my turn to be served.

'What can I get you?' the server asked.

'Ham and tomato sandwich, please.' I paused, then went for it. 'And a piece of coffee and walnut cake.'

'No problem.'

'And a doughnut.'

Chapter Eight

It was a couple of days later that I discovered more about the prisoner Pastor Clive had been so concerned about. His name was next on the ledger and I saw that he was 24 years of age. I went to the door to call him in and noted the stoop that Pastor Clive had mentioned. He was right, the young man was considerably hunched.

As he entered my room I could see that he was really nervous – he kept knitting his fingers together, pulling them back and yanking at them. When he sat down his leg was constantly jittering (and how that brought Kofi Aboah back to mind, that bouncing leg, not because of nerves but because of pain). He was certainly extremely thin. His head was completely shaved and I spotted a couple of sore patches where he'd fretted at a spot and made it bleed. Those nerves again; this was a man who couldn't be still.

'Hello, Aaden, it's nice to meet you,' I said. 'How can I help you?'

'The pastor,' he replied, his English awkward and broken. 'He make me.'

'Ah,' I said, nodding, 'yes, he did talk with me briefly about you, because I know he is a bit worried about you. So, tell me about your symptoms?'

He looked confused.

'How are you feeling? Have you become thin?' I asked, trying to keep the language simple and straightforward.

'Yes, I lose much weight,' he said. 'And sweat when sleep. Sweat a lot. But pain too much in back.' He pointed behind him. 'Much pain.'

I continued to work my way through enough questions to try to get a decent history.

'Do you mind if I examine you?' I asked, once we were finished. I needed to get a good look at his back

He nodded his agreement and we both stood up.

I noticed that there was a slight curvature of his spine which was the cause of his stooped posture.

I turned him around and gently pressed up and down his spine to see if there was any localised tenderness, and he winced when I reached his lumbar spine.

'Does it hurt here?' I asked.

He nodded.

'Could you lie on the couch for me?' I asked, pointing over to the examination couch. He did so and I checked to see whether he had any sign of pressure on his nerves. Fortunately, he didn't. I realised he was shivering – cold or nerves?

'Okay,' I said, gesturing towards my desk. 'That's all I can do for now, please take a seat again.'

We both sat down.

'Well, Aaden,' I said to him. 'I need to do some tests to be able to treat you properly, so is it okay if I arrange for you to have some blood taken?'

He nodded again but said nothing.

'You will also need to have a scan of your back and a chest X-ray at the hospital, which I will organise for you.' He was so quiet, tugging at his fingers over and over again. I needed to get across to him that it wasn't as bad as he clearly feared. 'As soon as we know what's wrong,' I continued, speaking as simply as I could, 'we can put it right.'

He continued to stay silent for a while and then quietly asked, 'I will die?'

'No, Aaden definitely not!' I told him. 'I think you may have an infection of your back that can be treated once we know for sure what's going on.'

He stared at me for a moment, his brain slowly accepting this new information. Then the emotion flooded from him, he broke down in tears, shaking and sobbing. 'Thank you, thank you, thank you … ' he sobbed. 'I been so frightened.' He looked so small and frail hunched up on the seat, rocking gently. We sat quietly together for a moment, just letting all the nerves and fear drain away. For a long time – perhaps months – he had been sitting on this condition, worsening and worsening, his terror building, his imagination firing. Like so many of the patients I had seen in the prisons I had worked in, they were prisoners of their own minds above and beyond the four walls that contained them.

The Devil's workshop! I heard Daniel Kobe's voice in my head and imagined him, twirling his mop and bowing.

'It's going to get sorted,' I told Aaden. 'And we are all here to help you. Especially Pastor Clive.'

'He is good to me,' Aaden nodded. 'I would not be here but for him.'

'He's a good man and a credit to the prison,' I agreed. 'Now, I'm going to prescribe you some painkillers and book an appointment with the nurse for you to get some blood taken, is that okay?'

He nodded.

'And then we'll see each other again in a few weeks, to see how you're getting on.'

'Thank you, Mrs Doctor,' he said. 'You been kind to me.'

He shuffled off, standing slightly straighter than he had when he came in.

*

I called in the next patient, a 32 year-old man from Zambia, called Jean-Luc Wakabi. As he took his seat, I couldn't help but notice that he looked remarkably fit.

'You clearly make use of the prison gym,' I said.

He smiled and rubbed, rather self-consciously, at his close-cropped hair. 'I would go mad, I think, if I weren't able to lift weights and work out in the gym. That's what keeps me going in here. The challenge to get fit gives me such a buzz. I love it. Trouble is, I think it's also what has caused my problem.'

'Oh'– I leaned forward – 'and what's that?'

He rubbed his chest. 'I've found a lump just here, that doesn't seem to want to go away. Can I show you?'

'Of course.'

He pulled off his tracksuit top and then his T-shirt while I pulled on a pair of disposable rubber gloves in order to examine him.

He felt around his chest to locate it.

'Ah. Here it is,' he said, poking it so that I could find it. 'I feel a bit embarrassed in case you think I am making a fuss about nothing,' he continued, 'because it's very small. The problem is I have too much time to think about things in here, and small worries get magnified into much bigger worries.'

The Devil's workshop – always the Devil's workshop.

I examined the lesion which was located on the anterior aspect of his right chest wall, and measured approximately three centimetres in diameter. It was smooth, soft, and didn't feel as if it was attached to the underlying muscle. *So far so good*, I thought.

'How long has it been here?' I asked.

'About three months,' he said. 'It doesn't hurt,' he continued, shrugging, 'so I figured it would just go away, but when it didn't, I decided that perhaps I should get it checked. So here I am.'

He smiled, but I could see that there were nerves beneath all this confidence.

'Well,' I said, 'it feels innocent enough and is almost certainly nothing to worry about. It actually feels like a fatty lump called a lipoma, but it's important to get it checked properly.'

He shrugged again. 'I presumed I'd torn a muscle in the gym. Wouldn't be the first time.'

'Yes, it may well be that, trauma can sometimes also cause lipomas, but usually they just appear for no reason. Do you remember any injury to your chest?'

He shook his head. 'No. And, actually, I am sure I would remember if I had.'

'You say that,' I replied, 'but sometimes people can be unaware of small injuries when they work out. Besides, if you work out a lot you may just have forgotten.'

He shook his head. 'My memory is … ' He tried to think of the right word. 'Strange! I rarely forget anything. Honestly. I'm an accountant, I think it comes as part of the job.' He tapped his head and grinned, a beautiful, joyful smile. 'This is a calculator. Or a camera! It all sticks. Honestly, nothing happened. I just noticed it one morning.'

'And has it changed size at all since you first noticed it?'

'No.'

'And it doesn't hurt?'

'Not at all.'

I removed my gloves and sat back down at the desk.

'All right,' I said. 'As I say, I'm sure it's nothing to worry about, but it's important to get it checked properly, so I'll arrange for you to have an ultrasound scan.'

'A scan? At hospital?' There was that big grin again. 'Great! I'm going on a trip!'

'With at least a couple of officers, I'm afraid,' I said. 'So don't get too excited.'

'You joking? I don't care if the whole staff come with me. Just to get a change of scenery, bit of a drive – brilliant, thanks, Doctor.'

I smiled back at him. 'You're welcome. I'll see you again after your scan.'

'Just name the date, I'll be there. I can't wait!'

*

The next patient was a young Bulgarian man who I had arranged to see.

I'd met him on my first day at Huntercombe, and on that occasion he needed help with a shoulder injury, and had been pleasant enough to deal with.

Bogdan Kolev was 26 years of age, and had been in the UK for eight years. When he'd first come over he'd been working as a labourer, but then a fight and a manslaughter conviction saw him remanded in the Young Offender Institute HMP Isis, and transferred to HMP Belmarsh shortly thereafter once he had been sentenced. Now he was in Huntercombe, prior to his deportation, with just under two years left to serve.

He had been diagnosed with latent TB during his last couple of months at Belmarsh, and was completing a three-month course of Rifinah, isoniazid and pyridoxine when I met him. He told me that he was very shocked and upset when he was informed that he had TB, especially as he was entirely asymptomatic.

On transfer to Huntercombe, he had been screened – as all prisoners are – for hepatitis and his hepatitis B core antibody was found to be positive, so I needed to discuss this with him.

'Hello, Mr Kolev,' I said.

'Good morning, Doctor.'

His manner was very formal and he had a rather severe and expressionless face. He behaved almost as if the consultation was an interview for the most important, the most daunting, job in the world. He sat ramrod-straight in his chair, his posture almost military.

I found myself wondering what life had been like for him back in Bulgaria, what his parents were like, what it was that had driven him to our shores when still only a teenager. Had it been a need for work, as it is with so many? Or was he running from something?

I hoped it was the former, as it was always hard to think of people being sent back to a country where danger might be waiting for them.

'As you may know,' I said, concentrating once more on the present, 'we screened you when you arrived here for hepatitis.'

He nodded.

'Well,' I continued, 'I arranged to see you today to let you know that the results show that you have positive antibodies for hepatitis B.'

He leaned forward, looking even more serious, and actually a bit threatening.

'I have hepatitis?' he said, almost accusingly

'Possibly,' I replied. 'But it is important to do some more tests to assess it further, as the results could equally indicate that you have *had* hepatitis B and it's now resolved, or that you have low-level chronic hep B infection. The results are negative for hepatitis A and C, so that's good.'

'Good?' he muttered, starting to rock backwards and forwards in his seat.

'Yes,' I continued. 'We need to do another blood test to check your liver function, and the lab have advised that we repeat the hep B tests so as to clarify things a bit further. As I said, it's entirely possible that you *had* an infection and it has resolved. Are you aware of any symptoms? Any loss of appetite? Nausea? Fever?'

'I could die?' He was shaking even more violently now as the impassive and formal façade began to crack.

'No, Mr Kolev,' I said, trying to keep my voice as calm as possible. 'In fact, a lot of patients with hepatitis B don't even need any treatment. They get over the infection within a few months. But, if needs be, it *can* be treated, so there's no need to get worried.'

I leaned forward, trying to lessen his anxiety as he was

obviously terrified. I wanted to calm him down as quickly as possible.

'What if it doesn't go away?' he said. 'Then what will happen?' His voice was getting louder and louder. 'Then what will happen?' He was almost shrieking now, beyond reason and clearly no longer listening to anything I was saying. He started shaking his head. 'I do not understand, how can I have this? Where has it come from? What have I done wrong?'

'It can be contracted in a number of different ways,' I said. 'And it doesn't mean you've done anything "wrong". It can be transmitted through sex, or shared needles, sometimes from tattoos. Do you have any tattoos?'

'I am not a drug addict!' he shouted, his fingers gripping at the legs of his tracksuit, pulling and yanking the fabric. 'I do not use needles!'

'I'm not accusing you of anything,' I insisted, keeping my voice as calm and level as I could. 'I am just trying to answer your question.' I was beginning to feel a bit irritated and almost angry myself.

'You're saying I am drug addict!' Suddenly he jumped up out of his chair.

'I'm not saying that, Mr Kolev,' I replied, as he towered over me. 'Can you calm down? I really need you to try to calm down ...'

'Calm down?!' he screamed at the top of his voice. 'You tell me I have this ... this disease ... and I am to be calm?'

I was beginning to think that I may need to press the

panic button when the door opened and a young officer called Luke came in. I have to admit I was very relieved to see him. Much like Mr Wakabi, Luke enjoyed the benefits of the gym. In fact, he made quite an intimidating sight as he walked slowly towards Mr Kolev.

'I heard a lot of shouting,' he said as he advanced, 'and wondered if you needed some help, Doctor Brown. What's going on?'

'She tell me I'm dying!' Mr Kolev screamed, and then it was as if the previously prim young man turned into a wild animal. He picked up the chair he'd been sitting on and swung it above his head. I couldn't say what it was he had planned on doing with it, as Luke moved too quickly for any of us to find out. He grabbed the chair with one hand and Mr Kolev with the other. Mr Kolev, still screaming, became utterly wild, spittle flying from his mouth, arms and legs thrashing as Luke pinned him to the floor. Fortunately, another officer heard the noise and came in to help. Within seconds the officers had restrained him and put handcuffs on him.

In those few minutes his demeanour had changed from calm and polite to completely frenzied. It reminded me of the only time I had ever pressed the panic button in Wormwood Scrubs, late one night in the First Night Centre. I had been chatting quite normally for a while with a prisoner who had just arrived in the Scrubs, when he suddenly leapt out of his chair and started banging his head over and over again on the brick wall. He was beating it so hard that I thought he was going to crack his head open and possibly turn on me and beat me up as well. Then, as now, the situation had been safely defused.

Mr Kolev was marched out of the room to the sound of cheers from the waiting room. A bit of drama to enhance the day never went amiss in a prison. There was nothing the prisoners liked more than a bit of a cabaret. The days were monotonous – any sign of excitement, of something different, would get a roar of approval.

Saroj appeared at the adjoining door. 'Are you okay?' she asked. 'Yes, I'm fine thanks,' I replied, but in truth I was actually feeling a bit dizzy because my heart was racing so fast. I took a couple of deep breaths. I knew, realistically, that the chances of anything *really* bad happening were minimal because, in a prison, help was always on hand. If need be, I could also insist on a chaperone for Mr Kolev's follow-up appointment, although I suspected that next time his behaviour would be different as he would have had time to calm down and process his thoughts.

Times like those always reminded me of some advice my husband David gave me many years ago. He said that if someone starts shouting and tries to pick a fight, if you don't react at all and just say nothing, they usually calm down because they realise that there's no point shouting at someone who doesn't shout back.

On the whole his advice has served me well over the years, which is a relief as I'm useless when I get angry. I can never think of the right thing to say at the time. It's usually a few hours later, when it's all over, that the best replies occur to me – when I've had a chance to calm down and process my thoughts. As a doctor, adrenaline can help me do my job, but it certainly never helps me win any arguments.

Thankfully, such occurrences are relatively rare. In general, the men know that I am there to help them, not to judge or punish them. They have no real reason to get angry with me.

The rest of the morning passed without any further surprises.

Chapter Nine

HMP HUNTERCOMBE
11 FEBRUARY 2014

At lunchtime I decided to pop over to the Rolls Inn. I was in the mood to treat myself to another lovely piece of freshly baked cake and a decent cup of coffee. I had a lot of correspondence and pathology results to go through, so convinced myself that I deserved it. Any old excuse!

Cutting across the courtyard, I was soothed by a gentle breeze that stirred the leaves around my feet as I walked. The weather had warmed up over the last few days and being outside no longer felt like an endurance test. The chill that seemed to graze the exposed skin had become a soft freshness that felt as if it held a little hope of spring, which really lifted my spirits.

A small group of men were walking back together from their various morning activities. Heading to their wings to have lunch. Chatting and laughing easily with each other. Behind them, walking on his own, I saw Usama.

'Doctor?' he said, noticing me. I stopped as he started to

walk towards me. His forearms were bound and he walked with that same hunch he'd had when I first met him. Folded in on himself, as if wishing he could just curl himself up into a ball and roll away out of sight. A man who wanted to leave no impact on the world. A man who ...

I shouldn't be here.

Well, yes, a man who knew what it was like to feel he had no place to be.

'Hello, Usama,' I said, as he caught up. 'How are you? I haven't seen you for a while.'

He shrugged, scratching slightly at his bandages. 'No, but I just wanted to say thank you.' He didn't meet my eyes, his gaze constantly low, staring at the dead leaves that spun around our ankles. 'You were very kind to listen to me.'

'I enjoyed listening to you, Usama,' I said, 'but I just felt so useless that I couldn't really do anything to help you.'

He nodded, a move so slight I almost didn't notice. 'I know. The nice people all say they feel useless. Because what can you do? How can you make it all right?' He let his words hang in the air for a moment. He knew there was no answer to them, certainly not yet. In time, perhaps, things would improve. But that time was, I feared, a long way off.

'It was good to be able to talk with you and not feel ashamed of who I am,' he continued after a moment. 'That is quite something. That is rare in my life.' He gave a weak, skimmed-milk smile, the best he could manage. 'You are very kind. Many people, they don't want to even listen.'

There was a pause for a moment, silence between us, and my heart felt heavy with the weight of his sadness.

'Is there anything I can do to help, Usama?' I asked, sensing that there was something here, some huge unspoken thing hovering between us. 'Anything at all?'

More silence. Then he shook his head, again a move so slight it was barely a move at all. 'I ... ' He hesitated for a moment. 'No,' he said in the end, shaking his head again, this time with considerably more force, more certainty. 'Thank you, there is nothing.'

He walked away.

I watched him for a few seconds, that hunched, thin frame, hugging himself, turned into an ill-defined silhouette against the sun reflected in the library windows. Not for the first time I tried to imagine his passage over here, the effort he had taken to escape the horrors of home. The determination, no ... the *desperation* that saw him accept any risk as worthwhile, anything to get away from the fighting, from what must have seemed the certainty of death.

Then to lose his partner.

I couldn't know how close they had been, not really, but sometimes a person's presence, their importance, can be defined by the space where they no longer are. To see Usama, to hear how he talked about Elias, was to understand the depth of love that had been lost. I thought of my husband David, and how much I loved him and relied on him every day. He was always there for me, when I needed to vent, to release the frustrations of my day.

He was there for the joy too, the successes, those many moments in everybody's life when you can make a difference to someone else's.

I thought back to how we first met.

*

I was 26, by which time I had quite resigned myself to the fact that I was unlikely to ever find someone I loved enough to spend the rest of my life with. I had convinced myself that I was destined to be alone and single all my life.

My experience in relationships up until then hadn't been positive, to the point where I was quite sure I would never be able to entirely trust a man. Obviously, everyone is different and I understand that it might seem unfair to think all men would be untrustworthy, but I had become so distrustful of men that most new relationships were doomed before they even had a chance to get started.

My sister met the love of her life when she was 16 and, fifty-three years on, she is still happily married. She would often try to fix me a date with anyone she hoped might be suitable, but they never were. It just didn't happen, so I was determined to make a happy independent life for myself, and not rely on anyone else for my happiness.

My favourite song at the time was Gloria Gaynor's 'I Will Survive'. It seemed to sum up my life, and I sang along to it, badly, whenever I heard it on the radio.

I had made my peace with a future of being alone.

But life had other plans.

By the end of January 1981, I had completed the final part of my training and was fully registered with the General Medical Council having finished my junior house jobs. I then spent the next six months as a senior house officer in Psychiatry at Wexham Park Hospital, in Slough. It was a department I knew only too well after spending my summer holidays working there as a cleaner back in 1973.

I had managed to secure a place on a three-year GP training scheme, based in Heatherwood Hospital in Ascot, which was due to commence in August, so I decided it was time to try to get on the property ladder. I was clearly going to be in the Ascot area for a few years and needed somewhere to live. Fortunately getting a mortgage back then was far easier than it is now.

But, however easy getting a mortgage offer might have been, actually *finding* somewhere I could afford and, more to the point, imagine living in, proved to be much more difficult. Eventually, in Bracknell, just down the road from the hospital, I found a small flat that fitted the bill. It was a new build, bright and modern, but after completing the deal in April, there was a small snagging list of problems that needed sorting out.

I contacted the developer and arranged to meet the man who was handling after-sales issues at the time.

As it took about forty-five minutes to get from Wexham hospital to the flat, I had to take a half-day's annual holiday in order to keep the appointment.

I arrived early, as I always do, and began to wait for the builder. And wait. And wait. And wait. As the time passed, sitting in this empty, unlived-in flat of mine, I became quite convinced that he wasn't going to arrive. I'd wasted a precious half-day of leave and would have to use up another half-day in the near future when the appointment was rescheduled. I was, in all honesty, furious. I gathered my things, put on my coat and went to leave when, just as I was about to open the front door, the doorbell rang. I opened the door, in a rage, and stared at the handsome stranger on the threshold.

'I'd just about given you up!' I told him.

As obvious as my anger was, he didn't react, but just looked at me, his kind beautiful eyes saying more than any words could. He was completely calm – wouldn't he later give me advice for this very situation? Never react with anger if presented with it! – and I felt a strange, soothing sense of that same calmness spread through me.

Little did I know then that I was looking at the man I was going to spend the rest of my life with. We went on a few dates. And slowly, gently, cautiously, I fell in love. I couldn't help myself, even though I was terrified of getting hurt.

*

Poor Usama.

The thought of what he was going through was heart-breaking and, as I continued on my way to the Rolls Inn, my head was miles away, imagining dangerous sea crossings and murderous drug gangs, all the things that I – like most of us – have never had to consider might threaten my life, or the lives of those I loved.

I ordered a coffee and a piece of chocolate cake, and while I was waiting, I saw the boss marching towards me along the corridor.

'Hello, David, how's things?'

'All good, thanks, living the dream as everyone says in here!' He clapped his hands with enthusiasm, rubbing them together. 'I'll be better when I've had something to eat though. My stomach's rattling I'm so hungry. I might even treat myself to a piece of that cake, as I don't think my usual baguette will touch the sides!'

The server handed me my cake and coffee.

'Actually,' said David, 'I'm glad I bumped into you today as I was going to ask if you might be able to help me on Friday, if you're free at lunchtime.'

'Of course. What's happening on Friday?'

'Our mutual friend, Mr Aboah,' he explained. 'I've actually managed to schedule a video call for him to see his wife.'

'Amazing! You must have had to jump through a few hoops to organise that.'

'I'd love to take all the credit, but I have a nagging suspicion I had a little extra help.'

'Oh?'

'Our VIP on Mountbatten,' he said. 'Mr Kuti?'

'Really? So he may actually have turned out to be a good new friend to Kofi after all.'

'I can't imagine Mr Aboah had anything to offer in return,' David agreed. 'So let's assume it's just a lovely piece of altruism. Anyway, it's scheduled for Friday.'

'Wonderful news! So, what can I do to help?'

'I'm aware that this is likely to be an extremely emotional time for Mr Aboah, and I'd feel more comfortable if there was someone from Healthcare on hand, just in case. Bit of moral support if nothing else.'

'I'm sure that won't be necessary.'

'Probably not but, well, wouldn't you like to be there? You've been of such great support to him.'

'If Mr Aboah has no objection then, of course,' I said, 'I'd love to be there.'

'Excellent,' said David. 'There's no time difference between the UK and Ghana, thankfully, so it was relatively easy to schedule. It's one o'clock. Can you manage that?'

'Definitely,' I said. 'How exciting!'

David took the baguette he'd ordered and gestured with it. 'Don't forget to bring some lunch. I'll make the coffee.'

Chapter Ten

OUT OF HOURS WORK
2006

I was once told about prison work: 'Doing a good job here is like wetting yourself while wearing a dark suit. You get a nice warm feeling but nobody else notices.'

It's not just in prison that doctors wear that dark suit.

One of the hardest jobs I've ever done is working for the out of hours GP service.

I was splitting my time between working in Huntercombe – my initial time there, when it was still for young offenders – and Salisbury, working on the end of life project and staying in a B & B for two nights of the week as it was too far to commute. It was affiliated with the Buckinghamshire hospital trust project with Stoke Mandeville and Wycombe hospitals.

In addition, I also worked for the out of hours service in Buckinghamshire – picking up shifts as and when I could fit them in.

The toughest one was the mobile 'red eye' shift which

began at eleven o'clock at night and finished at eight o'clock the following morning. The incoming calls were triaged by the doctor at the base and any patients needing a visit were passed on to the 'mobile' doctor out and about in the car.

On one occasion I had a message to phone a patient from the car as the base doctor could make no sense of what she was saying and was concerned.

'Need visit.'

The voice was so muffled, so slurred, I could barely understand.

'No problem,' I replied. 'But first of all, can you give me your address, please?'

'Lev … Lev … Levuh …'

'Eleven?'

'Mhuh. Levuh. Ladbruh … bruk … Ladbruk …'

The catchment area was absurdly vast, but there was a Ladbroke Road that had a truly wonderful Chinese takeaway on it. I'd built up my reserves with a tray of their mushroom chow mien on a number of nights.

'Ladbroke Road?' I asked.

'Mhuh.'

'Can you tell me what the problem is please?'

There was a slurred sound in reply, a low groan that made little sense. I looked to my driver for the night, Phil, who could tell that I was having some difficulty in understanding. He pointed at the road and shrugged, wondering if he should get going. I thought about it for a moment and then nodded, giving him the address, which he tapped into his satnav.

'Can you hear me?' I asked. 'I need to know what's going on.

Are you in pain? Can you br.....'

'Nevver muh ...' said the voice before I could finish trying to gather a few facts 'All fye ... dunt nee vizz ... dunt nee ... '

She hung up.

'Any clues?' asked Phil.

'I'm pretty sure she was saying she didn't need a visit after all,' I replied.

'What do you reckon then, Doc? Want me to carry on?'

I thought about it. It's not as if the service was undersubscribed – I needed to ensure that our time was well spent, emergency calls only. But that slurred voice ... It could have been down to so many things, and what if the woman really was in a bad way? She must have had sufficient cause to call in the first place, or believed she had.

'No,' I decided. 'Keep going.'

He nodded. 'No problem.'

Phil was one of my favourite drivers. His main job was working for the Fire Service and just occasionally there was a vague smell of smoke clinging to his clothes. He was doing extra shifts as a driver because he and his partner had a baby on the way and nothing sharpened the focus on the monthly bank statements more than that. I remember trying to help him one night as he searched on his phone for car seats, just before our shift started. It was lovely to see how excited he was at the thought of the new arrival who would bring so much love and joy into their lives.

Phil was muttering to himself as he continued to search his phone.

'Most of these look like they're designed for stoned gamers,' he said, turning the phone towards me. 'Look at that thing, all red and black and go-faster stripes. I want our baby to be a safe passenger, not up here thinking she's playing *Grand Theft Auto*.'

'She?'

He blushed a little. 'We wanted to know and were told at the last scan,' he said, clearly delighted.

I didn't envy life for his partner, stuck on her own all night while Phil was out here driving too quickly down B roads (or 'cow paths' as he insisted on calling them) trying to get me where I needed to be. I hoped he would cut down on his shifts once the baby was born

'Jenny and I have talked about it,' he'd said one night, after we'd discussed it. 'But she's okay on her own and sleeps quite well when I'm not there.' And then he laughed.

'I also snore like a pig singing thrash metal, always have. At least if I'm out here she's getting the rest she needs. Let's be honest, we won't be getting much in six months' time.'

That was likely true enough. Babies have no regard for whether their worn-out parents need to sleep or not. They enjoy working to their own schedule. Much like some patients during the red-eye shift on occasions, for that matter.

Babies can cry and have everyone running around just because they've wedged their soother down the side of their cot mattress. I once had a patient try to get me to visit because she couldn't reach the TV remote control from where she was sitting.

'I'm recuperating,' she had insisted. 'Done me foot with a shopping trolley.'

I suggested shuffling that extra few feet would be good exercise. Luckily, I knew her well as she tended to call the out of hours service on a very regular basis, I think mainly because she was so lonely.

I hoped this call wasn't another timewaster.

Phil pulled up on the side of the road, wedging us between two parked cars with the sort of one-handed, steering-wheel-spinning air of casualness that he always had. I didn't think I was a bad driver by any means, but I always found myself slightly in awe of people like Phil, who seemed so plugged into their car that it moved as if part of them.

'Thanks, Phil,' I said, grabbing my bag. 'Fingers crossed I'm not wasting both our time.'

'Time is never wasted with Judith Krantz,' he said, pulling a battered paperback from the cubbyhole in the car door. His taste in novels always surprised me. 'The socialites of Manhattan await my happy attention.'

I got out, closed the door behind me and walked a little way up the street. The old-fashioned, yellow streetlights turned everything into the flat colour of egg yolk and shadow. It was hard to read the numbers from the street, but I finally found number eleven lit by the second-hand blue of a flickering TV screen leaking from its front window. The gate was tatty, its latch rusted so that it took no small effort on my thumb's part to get it to open. The front lawn was an explosion of dandelions surrounding a small child's scooter as if to gang up on it.

I pressed the doorbell but, not hearing any result, rapped on the balloon glass window of the door. Still there was no response. I knocked again, peering through the distorting glass at a bulbous and surreal front room, sofa undulating, TV light dripping. Had the slurred-voiced woman passed out? Was she in trouble?

I knocked once more, glancing over my shoulder towards the car and Phil, whose face was burrowed between the pages of his novel. He looked thrilled.

The door opened. A small boy of no more than six was standing there, wheezing deeply, little hand clutched at the chest of Teletubbies pyjamas in fierce, fire-engine red. The yanked fabric turned the baby face of one of the antennaed aliens into an angry cone.

He tried to speak but it was clear that, in the depths of what appeared to be an asthma attack, words were beyond him.

'It's okay,' I said, 'I'm a doctor and I'll soon make your breathing better again. Is it alright if I come in?'

He nodded and I stepped inside, leading him to the foot of the stairs just a few feet from the door. 'Is your mummy about?' I asked, looking around, but he sat down on the stairs and just shrugged. What an answer that was. To be so young, in such a panic and simply not to know, to shrug, as if the absence of his mother was so commonplace as to require no more than a dismissive twitch.

'Wait here,' I said. 'I'll be straight back.'

I rushed back to the car, grabbed the nebuliser and quickly set it up so that he could breathe in the vaporised medication to open up his airways. Gradually his breathing began to ease and I tried not to think about the possible outcome of such a severe attack had I not been on his doorstep. When the nebuliser had completed its job, I removed the little mask from his face.

'What's your name, young man?' I asked.

'Martin,' he mumbled.

'Okay, Martin,' I said. 'Let's go and find your mummy, shall we?' I took him by the hand and we walked along the hall towards the front room and the flickering TV.

A movie was playing on the screen. Val Kilmer was pretending to be blind but Mira Sorvino still loved him. How good of her.

I saw a dark shape half-on, half-off the sofa.

'Can you just stand here for me, Martin?' I asked, fearing the worst.

He nodded and I left him in the doorway, trying to appear calm as I moved over to the body of his mother. I dropped to my knees to examine her and was hit by the sweet smell of white wine. On the floor there was a large bottle of Viognier half-wedged under the sofa. A fingerprint-smeared glass had a lipstick print brighter than the little left on her lips.

'What's your mum's name, Martin?' I asked, once reassured that her breathing was steady.

'Gina,' he said, his voice barely audible over Val Kilmer's performance on the TV.

'Can you hear me, Gina?' I asked. 'I'm the doctor you spoke to earlier. Do you remember calling me?' I gave it a moment then, louder: 'Gina? I need you to wake up now please Gina.'

Gina moaned slightly and her legs rolled off the sofa to join her torso on the floor. She mumbled a contented string of inaudible words, drew her legs up into her chest, a child sleeping in the foetal position, and began to snore. I sighed.

'Gina! You can't sleep anymore, I'm afraid, I need to be able to talk to you.'

'Tire …' she mumbled and pushed me away.

'I know you're tired, Gina,' I said, trying to keep my voice calm. 'So will I be by the end of my shift, I can assure you. Now, will you wake up for me?'

It took a further five minutes of cajoling and nudging but eventually I managed to get Gina sitting upright and showing some sign of consciousness.

'We need to get someone else round,' I said. 'Is there anybody you can call? I'm not leaving you here to look after Martin in this state.'

'He should be in bed,' she mumbled. 'Should be asleep.'

'Well, he's not,' I said, keeping my voice low. 'He's

standing over there trying not to panic about his mum. He's had a very severe asthma attack and needs to be in hospital to have regular nebulisers every few hours until he's better. Do you understand?'

Gina nodded.

'But I need to make sure there's someone else here who can keep an eye on you both until the ambulance turns up. Alright? So who can we call?'

'It's late,' she mumbled, looking at the clock on her phone. 'But I can try my mum.'

She made the call, while I led Martin through to the kitchen and poured him a glass of water from the tap.

I learned a long time ago that it is impossible to know how someone gets to wherever they are in life. I don't have the right to judge and for all I knew Gina may have been through hell. But, whatever hell she might have lived through, it was deeply upsetting to see how her behaviour was affecting her little boy. I waited until Gina's mother arrived, a short-tempered woman in black velvet pyjamas, who immediately swept Martin up into her arms and carried him upstairs to his bed to keep him warm until the ambulance arrived.

'She has issues,' the mum said as she passed, the sneer in her voice so pronounced it made me wince as much as the smell of spilled wine had earlier.

Back out in the car I discussed things with Phil. As was so often the way, the hardest thing sometimes for me was to accept the limits of my power to help.

'You were there for when the kid needed you, tonight,' said Phil.

'Yes,' I agreed, 'but what about tomorrow?'

*

The next call led us deep into the country, the streetlights left behind as we entered the thick coverage of trees and the high walls of hawthorn hedge. Phil's headlights swept to and fro as the road wound its way through the vegetation. Slicing through the leaves, shadows dancing, the lights searched for a sign of life, briefly reflecting in the eyes of a creature that fled into the undergrowth a fraction of a second after I'd registered it.

'These bushes,' said Phil, 'are the sort of bushes that murderous bastards leap out of.'

'Thanks for that, Phil,' I replied. 'They're just bushes.'

'You can't trust the country,' he said. 'Every horror film you see tells you. If you go to the country, they'll get you.'

'Who'll get you?'

'The nutters.'

'And which nutters would these be?'

'The sort of nutters that live in the country.'

I smiled, Phil was clearly not going to be dissuaded from his world view by anything as substantial as cold hard logic and actual facts.

'Watched a brilliant one the other night,' he continued. 'These two hired killers it was.'

'Oh yes.'

'Yeah. They go to the country though and, you know what happens?'

'Nothing good?' I guessed.

'Nothing good,' he nodded, forcefully. 'Precisely. Nothing good at all.' Then he grinned. 'It was brilliant. Have you seen the one with the Wicker Man ...? What's it called?'

Suddenly a deer bolted in front of us and Phil slammed on the brakes. The car stopped instantly, his reflexes as fast as always. I took a breath and rolled my neck, only too aware that it would tell me exactly how it felt about being whipped around soon enough.

'Sorry about that,' he said. 'Deer.'

'I saw.'

He smiled. 'Beautiful, wasn't it?'

'Beautiful,' I agreed feeling very relieved that the deer, Phil and I had escaped unharmed.

'Phil started the car again and pulled off slowly, clearly a little shaken. Eventually, we pulled up outside a small cottage. The upper walls were covered in ivy, as if the surrounding plant-life had decided to give the place a bearhug and then refused to let go. 'Do you want me to come in?' Phil asked, one hand already on the bowed spine of his paperback. 'Only the house is probably filled with psychos. Maybe even cannibals.' He laughed as he pointed at me. 'Nutters everywhere. Nothing good will happen.'

'You've definitely been watching too many stupid films.

I'm sure I'll be fine,' I said. 'If you hear me screaming, or frying in a pan for that matter, just come and rescue me.'

'Fair enough,' he smiled, cracking open his Krantz. 'Let's cross our fingers and hope for the best, shall we?'

'Let's.'

I walked up to the front door, my boots crunching on the gravel of the path.

The lights were on in the windows, but heavy curtains were drawn leaving thin gaps. As I knocked on the door I saw the flicker of movement, in the room to the left – someone running up and down, their shadow being thrown around behind them.

Whoever it was didn't come to the door but, after a moment, a small porch light came on and a stooped, elderly man appeared.

He opened the door. 'The doctor?' he asked.

'Yes,' I confirmed. 'I have come to see Jack Whiteside. Are you Mr Whiteside?'

He nodded. 'It's my son,' he said, his voice little more than a whisper. 'He's ... well, he's ...'

He appeared so nervous, glancing over his shoulder, even as a younger man suddenly appeared in the doorway behind him and pulled him, rather violently, out of the way.

'What's the problem?' the young man asked. The corners of his mouth were flecked with spittle, his eyes were wide, his hair on end as he kept running his hands through it, tugging it upwards. He suddenly turned and marched back into the house, still yanking at his hair. 'What's the problem? What's the problem?' he asked over and over again.

Well, yes, that was a good question, frankly.

I stepped cautiously into the house, looking to the old man. 'Are you all right?' I asked. 'Did he hurt you?'

'No, no, no,' he insisted, though his shirt was tugged from his waistband, one wing of the collar pointing up as if to flag a passing taxi. 'He wouldn't hurt a fly. Not really. It's just that he ... he gets a bit ...'

'What's the problem?' the young man shouted again, from somewhere else in the house, and I caught the sound of a woman's voice raised in panic.

'Now, Jackie!' she cried. 'Just have a sit down and we'll sort it all out. Don't we always sort it all out?'

'What's the problem?' he screamed.

I turned in the doorway and caught Phil's eye by waving. He tucked his book back in the door and climbed out.

'Problem?' he asked, walking over.

I looked to the old man who was still shaking his head, trying – and completely failing – to give the impression of a man totally at ease with the situation.

'Mr Whiteside's son appears to be having an acute psychotic episode,' I said to Phil, keeping my voice low. 'Best to be safe and go in together if you don't mind.'

'You think he might be violent?' he whispered.

'Possibly,' I admitted.

'Well then' – he gave a slightly nervous smile – 'I hope you're ready to protect me.'

We went inside and I could now see the young man was in the dining room that lay off the entrance hall. He was circling the dark wooden table in the centre of the room, his hand extended, fingers outstretched to touch the wood as he walked around and around. He was like a psychotic record player taking the highly polished mahogany for a spin.

'What's the problem?' he asked, again and again.

Jack suddenly broke away from the table, dashing past the woman I presumed to be his mother and running for the stairs.

'Oh, Jackie,' she sighed, resting a hand against her weary, sorrowful face. She was a big woman, and she had slightly wild, curly white hair. I couldn't tell if it was just unkempt, or whether Jackie had been tugging at it as much as he had his own. I hoped the former for her sake. She was wearing a floral-print dress and there was a dark spatter across the hem of the skirt.

'Are you all right?' I asked, moving over to her.

'Just tired,' she said. 'Ever so, ever so tired.'

'On your dress,' I said gesturing towards the large stain. 'Is that blood?'

Confused for a moment, she lifted the skirt up to her nose and then stared at it. I saw Phil, slightly embarrassed, turning away so that she wasn't exposing herself to him.

'Minestrone soup,' she said. 'From Sainsbury's. He's a posh boy, is our Jackie. Loves a spicy noodle. Oh, I'm so tired ...' She suddenly looked as if she was going to fall, so I quickly moved over to her to offer support.

'Phil?' I asked, not quite able to hold her on my own.

'I've got her,' he said, darting forward and grabbing hold as we managed to settle her safely on a chair by the table.

'Marj?' Her husband came running in. 'Has he hurt her?'

I shook my head, 'Not that I can see. I think she's just exhausted, with due cause I imagine.'

There was a sudden, terrifying crash from upstairs. Then a pounding that shook the ceiling, over and over again. The light above us, a dull bulb, began to shake, making the shadows dance in the room. I realised Jack was jumping on the beds.

'It's so difficult,' he said, gently stroking his wife's hand and saying her name. 'He looked up at me. We had him too late in life. That's what I think. He was always a handful. Always. He used to have me running up and down those stairs like Roger Bannister. So much energy.' He sighed. 'So much anger too.'

Jack started shouting again upstairs. 'What's the problem? What's the problem? What's the problem?'

'You should get on the phone, Doc,' said Phil.

'The phone?' Jack's father asked. 'It's a bit late, isn't it?'

It was both an absurd thing to say and also, strangely, completely on the nose. I had a feeling the mental health services should have been called a long, long time ago. It was clear that Jack would need to be sectioned and admitted to hospital for psychiatric care, but arranging for someone to be sectioned was invariably a lengthy process.

'Your son needs help,' I told him.

'Only on the bad days,' he said, his voice pleading. He

looked at his wife who was resting her head on her hands, her eyes closed. She mumbled something in her exhausted state. 'It'll break her heart if they take him away,' he said. 'Absolutely break her heart.'

She stirred, briefly, her eyes unfocused. 'It won't,' she said, her voice faint. 'It's what he needs. Me too.' She closed her eyes again. 'Then we can rest.'

I looked at Jack's father and tears were gently falling from his weary eyes.

'But what about my heart?' he asked. 'What about mine?'

Upstairs, Jack continued to bounce as I started the process that would keep Phil and I busy for the next hour or so. Even though I had managed to grab a couple of hours' sleep before the shift had started, I was beginning to feel really tired, but eventually, with all the arrangements for Jack sorted, Phil and I went back to the car.

*

Looking through the windscreen at the dawn breaking, sharing a flask of hot coffee with Phil, I tried to file away the many calls we'd handled before we set off again.

'Does this coffee taste of fish?' Phil asked.

I looked at him and took a sip of my drink. 'No,' I replied. 'It really doesn't.'

He sighed. 'Everything I drink tastes of fish at the moment,' he said. 'What's that all about?'

'Are you after a medical opinion?' I asked.

He looked at me, undecided and then nodded.

'Call the switchboard then,' I said with a smile. 'I'm due to clock off shortly.'

'Ha ha,' he moaned. 'Walked into that, didn't I?'

'In all honesty, I have absolutely no idea why you might be finding your drinks taste of fish. No idea at all.'

'And you went to doctor school and everything,' he announced with a smile.

'I did. Fully trained from "doctor school".'

He shook his head. 'Unbelievable.'

Another call came through. Phil looked at me and we both sagged in our seats at the thought of heading off on another visit so close to the end of our shift.

Half an hour later and we were pulling up outside a small, end-of-terrace house. As I got out of the car a man wearing a pair of overalls passed by.

He was wheeling a broken bike along the pavement, its front wheel bent horribly out of shape. He yawned and then said.... 'Rode straight into a kerb, didn't I? Half asleep, I was.'

It occurred to me that he was lucky a kerb is all he ran into.

I went up to the front door of the house and rang the bell. The door was immediately answered by a worried woman.

'Oh, thank goodness,' she said. 'You're the doctor?'

I nodded. 'Yes, hello, I'm Dr Brown.'

'It's our son,' she said, 'he's burning up with such a high

fever. We just don't know what to do. I'm so worried about him.'

She led me inside and up the stairs to a small bedroom, a universe of stars painted on the walls and a warm orange sun hanging from the ceiling.

'He wants to be an astronaut,' the father said, shaking my hand and sharing a worried look with his wife.

I moved over to the bed where the young boy slept.

'We took him to the doctor today,' the woman said. 'But he just said he had a virus. Told us to give him Calpol and plenty of fluids.'

I nodded and proceeded to examine him.

His cheeks were flushed and he had a very high temperature, but I couldn't find any localising signs to account for his fever, apart from the fact that his respiratory rate was slightly raised. He was also making very faint grunting noises, indicating that he might have a chest infection.

I just didn't feel happy with him and couldn't escape the fact that I had no choice but to send him to hospital.

"I think he needs to be admitted,' I told the parents.

'Admitted?' the dad asked. 'To hospital?'

I nodded.

I don't mean to worry you,' I insisted to the parents. 'I promise. I just want to rule out everything I possibly can.'

'His chest is clear though, isn't it?' the boy's mum asked. 'It was earlier. When the other doctor listened to him this morning.'

"Yes, it sounds clear but sometimes very young children's

chests can sound fine despite them having an infection. He is breathing a little faster than normal and making those little grunting noises. The only way to be absolutely sure is to have a chest X-ray,' I explained, 'as he may possibly need intravenous antibiotics.'

I got on the phone and contacted the paediatrician on call. It took some persuasion, but I eventually managed to arrange for the little boy to be admitted.

*

'Hello?' The voice on the phone sounded tired. I hoped that wasn't a bad sign.

'Hello, it's Doctor Brown. I visited the other night, to see your son?'

'Of course! Yes! We were just talking about you, actually.'

Oh God, nobody ever wants to hear that. Was I now the bane of all paediatric staff at Wexham Hospital? 'Oh yes?' I asked cautiously. 'Nothing too bad, I hope?'

'When we got to the hospital,' she continued, 'we insisted that they X-ray Josh. Like you'd said.'

'Right.'

'And they weren't going to do it. They just weren't. The doctor there listened to his chest and said there was no need. But we kept insisting,' she said.

'I'm afraid we might have been a bit of a pain actually.'

'I'm sure not. And?' I asked. 'Did they do it in the end?'

'They did and it was awful.'

'Awful?'

'A white-out, the doctor called it.'

Oh God …

'They transferred him straight to the specialist paediatric unit in Oxford.'

'Really?' I hardly dared ask. 'And? How about now … How is he doing?'

'He's getting there,' she said. 'Definitely getting there.'

I sunk with relief into my armchair – arms, back and legs reduced to liquid.

'Not out of the woods yet,' she continued. 'He's still having intravenous antibiotics but he's on the mend and the doctors are happy with his progress. It's been the worst few days of my life,' she said and started to cry.

When I put the phone down my mind felt numb for a few minutes, almost unable to process what I had just been told.

I decided there and then to never do another red-eye shift again.

I would never have forgiven myself if I hadn't managed to persuade the doctor on call to admit Josh that night. It was too dreadful to even contemplate.

My red-eye nights were over.

Chapter Eleven

HMP HUNTERCOMBE
14 FEBRUARY 2014

The sunlight falling through the window had all the warmth of a photograph of a snowman. Trust the heating in Healthcare to go on the blink the very morning the weather decided to return to the freezing temperatures of a few weeks ago.

'You might as well gather around a candle,' tutted Rosemary as she gave the plug in-heater she'd just turned on a gentle kick.

'Kicking it won't help, you know,' said Darren, the mental health nurse. Rosemary narrowed her eyes at him. 'Kicking things warms me up,' she said. 'Want to help me get toasty?'

Darren laughed but I could tell he wasn't entirely sure she was joking. He fiddled awkwardly at one of his ear piercings. 'Anyway,' he said, finally, 'I've got to get on.'

'Do,' said Rosemary, with a scary grin.

Darren shuffled off and Rosemary watched him go.

'He's terrified of you,' I said to her.

'Then he's as clever as his qualifications suggest,' she replied. 'I'm a menace. A loveable menace, but a menace nonetheless.' She laughed and then stomped off to her office, heels pounding out the usual drumroll on the hollow floor as she went.

It was the Friday of Mr Aboah's video call and I was feeling really excited about it. I tried to be warmed by the thought as I certainly needed all the help I could get; my room was freezing.

I sat down at my desk, overcoat wrapped tightly round me, and tried to warm my hands up on a large mug of coffee. They were white and numb with the cold.

I logged on and started checking through my routine lists. I had several pathology results back, including for Aaden, the patient Pastor Clive had convinced to come and see me. The tests showed that he had an elevated ESR and CRP ('erythrocyte sedimentation rate' and 'c-reactive protein'). Both of these tests are non-specific indicators of inflammation and can be raised due to anything from infection to cancer. The results certainly didn't surprise me because his history was highly suggestive of TB affecting his spine. Although rare, I had seen a patient in Wormwood Scrubs about a year previously with a very similar presentation, but sadly his disease had progressed further and had affected his spinal cord by the time it was diagnosed.

They were both from Somalia and similar in age.

The results of Aaden's scans and X-rays were not back

yet, so I would have to wait a little while longer to put the whole picture together. However, the result of Mr Wakabi's ultrasound scan *was* back, and I was really surprised to read that the lesion on his chest was thought to be suspicious. The report advised referring him for a biopsy and an MRI scan to rule out the possibility of a malignant tumour.

I was *definitely* not expecting that. I made a mental note to organise the referral at the end of the day, as it was already nearly time to start the clinic.

The first few patients were quite straightforward, and happily I didn't need to use the translation service for any of them, so for a change I was running more or less on time. Such a relief, as I didn't want to be late for the video call. However, the next man on the list was not quite so quick to deal with.

His name was Franciszek Kowalcyzk and, as with so many of the names, I had to practise pronouncing it before I went to call him in. I found it embarrassing that so many of the names were difficult for me to pronounce, and it was important to try and get it right.

He greeted me with a smile, which was always a good start, although he looked a little vague and as if he was slightly surprised to see me for some reason.

'Hello, Doctor.'

'Hello, Mr Kowalcyzk. What can I do for you today?'

'My cellmate, Karl, he is worried about me. He said I need to see you, but I think he's the one who needs to see you.'

'Oh. Why is that?'

'He snores and it is a real problem. A real, *real* problem.'

'For you or for him?' I asked.

'For me,' he replied. 'Because I can't sleep and it's driving me crazy, *and* for him because I think the only cure might be to kill him.'

There was a moment of silence.

'I can't help with your cellmate's snoring,' I explained, deciding to leave his other comment. 'Unless he chooses to come and see me.'

'Maybe I will help him by putting a pillow over his face, eh, Doctor?' He laughed. 'But let us hope it does not come to that.'

He smiled at me, as if to reassure me that it was a joke.

'So, back to you,' I said, very much wanting to get away from Karl's snoring. 'Why is Karl worried about you?'

'Because a few nights ago I was sitting on my bed and he said that I seemed to be completely out of it for about five minutes. I was dribbling apparently, and didn't realise that he was talking to me. It really spooked him out. When I came round he said that I didn't know where I was for a few minutes and seemed to be … what is the best word?' He looked up for a moment, as if hoping to find the word on the ceiling. 'Disorientated,' he decided. 'I was not aware of what had happened. Had no memory of it at all.'

'Do you know if you made any funny movements?' I asked. 'Bit your tongue or wet yourself.'

'No!' He recoiled in his seat. 'It would have freaked me out if I wet myself.'

'Has anything like this happened before?'

'I'm not sure, but I was stabbed in the head about five years ago and since then I've had times when I have felt a bit weird. I also get a lot of headaches.'

I was thrown for a moment. 'Stabbed in the head?'

'Yeah, with a carving knife. I got into this really bad fight back in Poland, but never went to hospital because I was on the run at the time.'

I had so many questions: Why? Who by? None of which were really medical in nature, I must admit. So many fascinating stories I will never get to hear, hiding behind the incredibly diverse collection of people I meet every day at work.

I looked at his notes briefly, but there was nothing of any significance.

'Well, the only way to find out why you had this weird episode is to refer you to the neurology clinic, and they can advise you what tests you need. Is that okay?'

'What kind of tests?'

'Most likely a brain scan, and also an EEG to look at the electrical activity of your brain. They just need to try to find out if there's any reason to explain your symptoms, and obviously recommend treatment if needs be. Very occasionally they suggest keeping people in for a period of observation, but I think that's very unlikely. You won't know exactly what they will suggest until you get there.'

He looked shocked. I thought he was overcome with fear at the thought of what might be wrong with him.

'But I can't go to hospital.'

'Why ever not?'

'Because I won't be able to smoke if I stay in hospital!' he said, as if stating the obvious. 'It's just not possible.'

I couldn't believe my ears. 'You'll refuse a hospital visit because they don't let you smoke?'

'Yes, absolutely, of course. Sorry for wasting your time, but I definitely don't want to go. I'll just have to put up with not knowing what's wrong with me. I'm sure it can't be that serious.' He stood up to leave. 'Thanks for your time, Doctor. Have a nice day.'

And off he went.

I felt drained and exasperated, and also very frustrated that the last twenty minutes had been a complete waste of time. *There's just no helping some people*, I thought, as I tried to brace myself for the next patient.

*

On and on the morning went, and just to add a bit more frustration to the day, I needed to use the translation service for a Russian and then a Portuguese prisoner. Eventually, when I had finished seeing the last patient on the list, I was free to go to attend Mr Aboah's video call. I was feeling nervous but excited at the same time.

'Doctor.' David nodded in greeting as I arrived at his office. 'We're set up in one of the conference rooms. Did you get a chance to pick up any food?' He held up a hand, stopping my reply. 'What am I saying? Of course you didn't, you hate to be late so you'll have come straight here.'

'Yes, bit of a heavy morning so I didn't have time. But it's not a problem, I can go without food for a change. It won't do me any harm.'

'You can share mine.' He tapped on a Tupperware box under his arm and gestured for me to walk ahead towards the conference rooms.

'That's very kind of you, but I don't want to steal your lunch, David,' I said as we walked along the corridor.

'You're not. I made extra because I thought you might skip lunch. You don't get to be Number One Governor of a prison like this without anticipating the worst, you know.' He smiled.

'If the worst today has to offer is a lack of sandwiches, I'll be over the moon,' I said. 'Though my morning's already had its fair share of stress.' I told him about the patient who was refusing to go to hospital because he smoked.

David shrugged. 'You can only help people who want it. That's one of the first things I think I learned doing this job. We all want to make people's lives better, that's what we're here for.'

We entered the conference room, the first to arrive. At the far end a chair had been set up at the table, facing a large laptop with a webcam plugged into it. We sat down and David popped the lid off his Tupperware box of sandwiches, sliding the box towards me so that I could take one.

'You know I told you about that programme I'm working

on?' he continued as we ate the sandwiches. 'Huntercombe Stories, where we follow some of the men who leave here and document their next steps, the decisions they make – hopefully with our support and assistance – that sees them making a fresh start.'

'I remember,' I said.

'Helping people who want it,' he continued. 'Because you have three types of people in a place like this: those who really want to change, those who might be convinced, or inspired to, and then, sadly … ' he tailed off.

'Those who will *never* change,' I finished for him.

He nodded. 'And you can spend so much time banging up against that, smacking your head against the brick wall of their personalities. Or … you can dedicate your time to helping those who really want and need your help. By supporting and documenting the first group, those who really want to change, and sharing their stories with the second group, those who can be convinced, who just need that little nudge, that proof that it can be done, that it's all worthwhile. Well … that's me doing the very best job I can do as Governor, I think. Beyond the day-to-day logistics of keeping everyone safe and fed, it's what we're all for. Talking of that, have you had a chance to see the training areas yet?'

'No,' I admitted, helping myself to another sandwich. 'Beyond what you showed me on the first day here, my life is restricted to Healthcare and the walk to Rolls Inn. I remember you mentioning them, though. A decorating course? Bricklaying?'

'And the craft centre, yes.'

'Oh yes, the hedgehog houses!'

David smiled. 'That's right. Have you bought one yet?'

'No.' I laughed. 'I have, so far, been a bit too busy to go and buy a hedgehog house, but I promise I will as soon as I can find the time.'

'Good. I'm sure you won't regret it and neither will the hedgehogs.' He smiled. 'Everyone needs a home.'

We chewed silently on our sandwiches.

'My point is,' he continued, after a moment, 'they're the heart of the prison. And the gardens, of course. It may sound like a cliché, but working hard at the soil, growing things, cultivating … it's such an obvious metaphor, really.'

'We want to help these men to grow.'

'Exactly. You have the last sandwich.' He pushed the box towards me.

'No thank you, I'm really full. Any more and you'll have *me* growing.' I looked at my watch. 'Shouldn't they be here by now?'

David glanced at his own watch and reached for the final sandwich. 'Any minute now,' he said. 'I always make a point of being early.'

'Quite right,' I agreed.

'Yes,' he smiled. 'But *I* do it to keep everyone on their toes, you do it because you're nice.'

At that moment a young man walked in with a laptop under his arm. He stopped in the doorway, looking slightly panicked. 'Am I late?' he asked.

'See what I mean?' said David, to me, grinning. He turned back to the young man. 'Please take a seat, Mr Salisbury, you're perfectly on time.'

'Oh.' The young man visibly relaxed, seeming to shrink a couple of inches. 'That's all right then.' He took a seat opposite us at the table.

'Mr Salisbury is one of our tech people,' said David.

'George, please,' the young man said, leaning across the table to shake my hand. 'You're Doctor Brown?'

'Yes,' I said. 'Very pleased to meet you. I'm sure my presence won't be needed but I am so happy to be here.'

'I wish I were,' he said in a bit of a grumpy tone. 'These things always sound well and good until the time comes, and then usually something goes wrong.'

'Maybe you should get set up?' suggested David. George nodded and shuffled over to the chair in front of the laptop and camera and started pressing buttons. After a moment the laptop sprang into life with its little singsong sound.

'You sound happy now,' George muttered to the laptop, 'but I bet you'll be in a mood soon enough.'

'Now, now, Mr Salisbury,' said David. 'Let's think positive, shall we?'

George shrugged. 'Computers are stupid.'

'You don't like them?' I asked. 'But surely ...'

'I work in tech,' he replied, 'so I must like computers? Oh, don't get me wrong, I *used* to like them. I liked them so much that I went to university and got a degree in computing. Now I work with them. And they hate me. Every day, they hate me. They won't turn on, they won't turn off, the screens cut out, they don't understand what the internet is anymore, they make strange noises, they won't make *any* noise ... Oh, trust me, computers are just the worst things, ever.'

I was a bit taken aback by his little rant but thought it best to say nothing.

He started tapping on the keys and muttering to himself.

David sighed. 'You'll have to forgive Mr Salisbury's enthusiasm,' he said, sarcastically.

Luckily, we were saved any further complaint from the IT department by the appearance of Mr Aboah. He was accompanied by one of the officers I had met on the tour with David.

'Thank you, Mr Holland,' said David, getting to his feet. 'How are you feeling, Mr Aboah?'

I could see only too clearly that Kofi Aboah was extremely nervous. I wondered how long it had been since he had seen his wife. He nodded gently, the swelling on his neck having got larger in recent weeks.

'I am excited, thank you, Governor.'

I stood up. 'Hello, Mr Aboah,' I said. 'Are you quite sure you don't mind me being here?'

'Of course not, Doctor,' he said. 'I would rather you were ... I feel a bit ...' His voice faded away as if he was unsure of how to put it into words. He thought for a moment and then settled on: 'I am nervous and my body will not let me forget. I can't stop shivering.'

'That's perfectly understandable,' I said. 'This is a really big day. How is the pain?'

Kofi tried to smile but he couldn't quite inject it with the good humour he was aiming for. 'It is getting worse,' he said. 'But the new pills are still helping a lot.'

'It might be necessary to alter the dose, so I will have a look at your notes this afternoon. I promise I will do my best to try to control your pain,' I said.

'Because that is all that can be done,' he replied and the weight of sadness in his voice pressed down on the whole room. For a moment, George stopped tapping. There was silence, all of us aware of the awful, irrefutable truth of what Kofi Aboah was facing.

'Sorry,' he said after a moment. 'I do not mean people to feel awkward. Some days are harder than others.'

'You have nothing to apologise for, Mr Aboah,' said David. 'I'm just glad that we might be able to bring you some happiness today.' He looked to George. 'Mr Salisbury?'

'Connecting now, sorry. It takes a minute to dial in to the secure server and establish a ...' his voice petered out as he realised that nobody needed to know the details right now. 'Well, anyway, be right there ...'

I stepped over to Mr Aboah and put my hand on his arm briefly.

'I'm sure the call will go really well and you won't be nervous once you see your wife again. This is a happy day for all of us.'

He tried to smile. 'Yes, I will be all right. I think. I hope.'

I could see the shivering, his whole body quivering with nerves. 'You should sit down,' I suggested. He nodded and I led him to the seat next to George who was speaking into the camera.

'Hello, this is George Salisbury, IT consultant at HMP Huntercombe, we have Mr Kofi Aboah here, very much looking forward to talking to Mrs Aboah.'

'Amba,' said Kofi. 'Her name is Amba.'

'Amba,' George added, rather weakly. 'Sorry.'

On the screen of the laptop I could see a man in a suit and tie sitting in a similar room to ours, albeit with the flag of Ghana visible in the background, its bright red, yellow and green stripes standing out cheerfully in what was, otherwise, a distinctly drab room.

The man's lips were moving but we couldn't hear what he was saying.

'Mr Salisbury?' David asked, having moved behind the IT technician. His tone was somewhat impatient, the last thing anyone needed in a moment like this was a technical problem.

'I think it's them,' said George, a slight edge of panic creeping into his voice. 'I really do think it's them.' He leaned towards the camera. 'Have you got your sound turned on?' he said in a slow, rather loud and deliberate manner.

'You're not talking to a dotty aunt,' David muttered. 'Shouting at it won't help anything.'

George went somewhat red. 'Sorry sir, yes sir.' He sat back a little and repeated. 'You may have to check your settings for the microphone. Can you hear us?'

Kofi Aboah moaned gently, his shaking getting worse. This whole situation was so stressful for him.

'I'm sure they'll get it working,' I said to him. 'Probably just a few teething problems.'

'Maybe it is better if it doesn't work,' said Kofi. 'Yes, maybe that would be best.'

'You don't mean that,' I said. 'I've seen how you look at the photo of your family. This is just what you and your wife need, a chance to reconnect.' I nearly added to that, nearly suggested that hopefully they would be able to do so face to face soon. I stopped myself. We really had no idea if David's plans to get Kofi home early would work. The last thing I wanted to do was give him false hope.

'You don't understand,' said Kofi. 'Amba hasn't seen me like this. Not with this so … ' He waved his fingers at the swelling on his neck. 'It is disgusting. Awful. She will be horrified by me. She will think I am … I am … I am …' He couldn't find the words but I could see the beginnings of tears in his eyes.

'She will think you are her wonderful husband,' I said. 'As if such a small thing as a swelling in your neck would put her off the man she loves. She will have missed you as much as you've missed her, you just see.'

Of course, I hoped I was right. I couldn't possibly know. Not really. All we had to go on was Kofi's side of the story.

Did we really know anything about this marriage? This family?

'… not here,' came the voice of the man on the computer screen. 'Can you hear me now?'

'Loud and clear,' said David. 'Though we missed what you said first. Someone not being there?' I could hear the concern in his voice and shared it – after all, there was really only one person whose absence was likely to be an issue.

'Amba Aboah,' said the man on the screen. 'She is not here. Not yet. It would seem there has been a problem with communication.'

Kofi moaned again, a low, guttural sound. The sort of sound we never really want to make, a pure venting as if a microphone had been held up to his very soul.

David cleared his throat, I could tell he was doing his very best to maintain his patience. 'Communication problem?' he asked. 'This call was booked some time in advance.'

'Not a communication problem with us,' the man on the screen said, rather defensively. 'With her. I was told she had been informed of the call but it now seems that she never received the message. Not to worry though. We are in contact now.'

'You're in contact with Mrs Aboah?' David asked.

'Yes,' said the man on the screen, quite happy to leave it at that.

David allowed a moment for the man to elaborate, but it seemed clear that he had no wish to. 'And?' David prompted. 'Where is she?'

'Shopping,' the man replied, again seemingly content with this one word answer.

'She's shopping?' said David.

'Yes,' the man replied.

'But she knows about the call now?' David asked and I noticed a quick, subtle glance towards Kofi. David was only too aware of how Kofi could be affected by all this. This was a man who was hanging on to life through sheer determination; the last thing he needed was to have that determination eroded.

'Yes she has just been informed,' the embassy man said, 'and she will be here as soon as is possible.'

David let out a long breath, utterly determined not to lose his temper. 'As soon as possible? Can we be a bit more specific than that?'

'She needs to find someone who can drive her to the embassy,' the man said.

'You couldn't send a car to pick her up?' David asked, unable now to keep the tone of incredulity from his voice.

'That is not our responsibility,' the man said, as if David were being quite ridiculous. 'It is more than we need to do that we have agreed to this call. It is a considerable imposition.'

'I appreciate that,' said David and I noticed his hand, gripping the back of George's chair as he leaned past the IT technician to look into the camera. His knuckles were quite, quite white. However he kept his tone even. 'Still, this is a – please excuse me Mr Aboah' – he glanced at Kofi before returning his attention to the camera – 'a dying man who wishes to speak to his wife. I'm sure we're all only too happy to bear a few slight impositions to make that happen, aren't we? After all … ' and here his voice really took on weight, 'we're all reasonable people, aren't we?'

'We are here, are we not?' the man on the screen said. 'And when his wife gets here, he can talk to her. Until then, what do you expect me to do?'

And with that, the man reached forward and cut the call. The screen went blank.

Kofi gave a wail of pain, both physical and emotional.

'Get them back, please, Mr Salisbury,' said David.

'He might not answer,' said George.

'Oh,' said David, 'he'll answer, because you're going to keep calling and keep calling until they have no choice. Aren't you?'

'Yes, sir,' said George, rather sheepishly.

'I'm sure they'll sort it,' I said to Kofi. 'You heard what he said. She's trying to get a lift to the embassy. I'm sure someone will be able to drive her, won't they?'

He was shaking his head. 'I don't know, I just don't know … ' Then a thought occurred to him: 'Maybe her cousin, she might do it. She works at night so she would be free.'

'Well,' I said. 'There you go then. See? You'll be chatting away soon enough.'

If only. While George kept hitting 'redial' on the screen, nobody was answering on the other end. David was trying not to pace, moving to the window and doing his very best to appear calm as he looked out through the blinds at the gardens outside. A small group of prisoners were working the soil. A couple of officers watched as the prisoners dug and turned the earth, plumes of condensed breath huffing from their mouths, clouds of effort. One of them strolled over to where a sapling lay on the ground, it's thick root bole shedding dirt as the prisoner picked it up to plant it. He placed the sapling in the hole they had dug together and held it while the other prisoner shovelled the earth back in.

'Just the job,' David muttered to himself, nodding with approval.

Time went on and the officer, Mr Holland was replaced by another, Mr Burton, who sat in the corner, patting his knees with impatient fingers and occasionally puffing out frustrated bursts of air.

'She is not coming,' said Kofi. 'I know that she is not.'

'She'll be there,' I tried to reassure him. 'Just give her a little more time.'

He was looking paler with every moment that passed, the stress and the nerves of the situation draining the little energy he had. There would come a point where I would have to say that, for his own health, we would need to give up and let him go back to his cell. But how could I make a call like that? Knowing what was at stake? Being a doctor often involves making difficult decisions but I had never faced one like this before.

I looked to David, knowing that he must be only too aware that time was running out for everyone. Regardless of what was at stake, we couldn't all just sit there indefinitely. We all had work to do. If I didn't make the decision to call it a day, he would certainly have to.

'They're still not answering, sir,' said George who had turned the volume down on the laptop as the repeated sound of the call ringing out was more than any of our nerves could stand.

'I'm aware of that, Mr Salisbury,' said David. 'Keep trying.'

George sighed but hit the button again.

'I remember,' Kofi suddenly announced, 'on our first date. We were going to a café. A good place, served excellent jollof and banku. I was so excited. I wouldn't show it, of course, because I was stupid. Trying to be the big man, you know? All swagger. All confidence. But she was the prettiest girl I had ever met. The prettiest. And she made me laugh so much. I was ...' He thought about the right word. 'I was intimidated by her, really. That is the truth of it. Scared of her. She was so much better than me. She deserved so much better. But instead of letting that show I tried to act cool. Stupid. Like I did not care. Like I wasn't sat there in this café, the smell of plantain, tomatoes, spice ... thinking that I was about to have the most important meal of my life. The most terrifying, amazing, beautiful bowl of rice anyone has ever had. And I waited. And I waited. And after a while it got difficult to look cool anymore, you know? Because people were looking at me. They knew I was waiting. They knew she was late. They thought she would probably not come. *I* thought she probably would not come! And I waited. And I waited. And now I am not cool, I am not cool at all. I am sweating, I am panicking, I am embarrassed, ashamed, but most of all, so, so sad. Because she was the prettiest girl I had ever met and she made me laugh. And I wanted so much to eat a meal with her. And somehow convince her that she might one day love me. Yes. That was the main thing. I wanted her to love me because, even when we arranged that very first date, I knew that I loved her.' He paused for a moment and sighed in pain, his leg shaking, his teeth clenched. I really would have to intervene; this was doing him no good ...

'And then,' he continued, 'just when I thought that I was going to have to just stand up and leave – walk out without having the most important meal of my life – she came in. She was hot, sweating, her blouse was torn, she had oil on her face and mud on her knees. When she came running over to me I could smell that bitter smell of electrical burning, of a gearbox that has died. She sat down, telling me all about what had happened. About how her scooter had broken down and of how she had had to walk it all the way here. She rubbed at her face and left even more dirt behind, two thick tracks of oil, all the way down her cheeks! And you know what? Covered in oil. In mud. Sweating, clothes torn. She was still the prettiest girl I had ever seen. And the best. And the cleverest. And the funniest and ...' He sighed again. 'She still is.'

Suddenly, the laptop screen came to life and George all but fell backwards off his chair.

'They're answering!' he said.

David sagged with relief. I knew he must have been about to call it a day. Now, hopefully, that decision would never have to be made.

'She is here,' said the brusque voice of the man who had previously hung up on us. With that he reached forward, his hand huge on the screen, and turned the camera so that it faced the woman sitting next to him.

She was obviously a little older than she appeared in the photograph I'd seen – and certainly the last few years can't have been easy for her, looking after the family on her own while the man she loved was kept away from her, dying in another country – but I was struck by how immediately recognisable she was, how deeply familiar from that totem of a photograph Kofi carried with him.

'Kofi? Are you still there?' her voice crackled, cutting out briefly.

All fear was gone from Kofi, that terror he had felt at being seen; he darted along the table, George jumping out of the way so that Kofi could take his seat in front of the laptop.

'I am here, my love, I am here.'

'Oh, Kofi …' There was a fragility to her voice, and I wondered how it must feel for her to see him. How much weight had he lost since she last saw him? How pronounced, how alien that growth must look.

'I think that perhaps …' David mumbled, standing up and ushering us all back from Kofi.

We couldn't leave him alone of course, sadly, but we did our best to respect the privacy of that moment, retreating to the doorway.

'I thought this was going to be a washout,' I whispered to David.

'You and me both,' he agreed.

While we did our best to ignore the call it was obvious from the occasional grating bursts of feedback that the quality wasn't all it might be.

'Maybe I should just …' George inched back towards Kofi and the laptop but David held his arm.

'Leave it, Mr Salisbury,' he said. 'They only agreed to five minutes and the last thing Mr Aboah will want is to spend half of that watching you fiddle with your damn settings.'

'Understood,' said George. There was a pause and then he couldn't help adding: 'The problem's probably their end anyway.'

'Are we any further ahead with plans to get Mr Aboah released?' I whispered to David.

He shook his head. 'I'm currently trying to find a doctor – an independent doctor, you understand, a second opinion if you like – to agree that it's likely Mr Aboah's condition will … ' He glanced at Kofi, clearly concerned about being overheard and pulled me slightly further into the corridor. It was probably unnecessary; Kofi was clearly utterly focussed on the video call – I think we could have shouted next to him and he still wouldn't have heard us.

'Sorry,' said David, 'just trying to be a little

circumspect. I need an oncologist to confirm that it's likely Mr Aboah will die from his illness before he gets released. But, of course, you know what these people are like ...'

I smiled. 'What people, David? Doctors?'

'Oh, I don't mean you,' he blustered. 'I just meant ...' He sighed. 'Nobody wants to state so definitively when Mr Aboah could die. There are too many variables and nobody is willing to stake their professional name on it.'

'It can certainly be very difficult to state, with absolute certainty, when someone will die of cancer,' I agreed.

'I understand that,' he replied. 'It just makes things so terribly difficult. Without someone going on the record to say that using the Early Release Scheme won't be quick enough ... I'm out of options.'

I nodded.

Back in the room it was clear that their conversation was coming to a close and slowly, respectfully, we moved back in.

'Thank you,' said the brusque man at the embassy. And the screen cut off. Kofi sat there for a moment looking at the black rectangle that had held his wife. He had tears in his eyes but the shaking had stopped, he was utterly still, transfixed even, by the computer in front of him.

'Sorry it couldn't be longer, Mr Aboah,' said David.

Kofi shook his head but still didn't speak.

I rested my hand on his shoulder. 'How are you feeling?'

For a moment he continued to stare at the screen and then, as if snapping out of it, glanced up at me. 'I need to hold on,' he said. 'Because I will see that woman again.' He nodded, a real sense of determination in his eyes, his jaw clenched. 'I will see all of them, I will hold all of them. I will look them right in the eyes and I will tell them two things. I will tell them that I am sorry, and I will tell them that I love them.' He looked right at me. 'I will do that,' he said. 'And nothing will stop me.'

Chapter Twelve

Every day I worked at Huntercombe, I was required to visit the segregation unit or 'Seg'.

It was just along the corridor from Healthcare, and consisted of five small cells where prisoners who either needed reprimanding or, perhaps, protection and close observation, were held.

I had been locked in one of the cells once, just to feel what it was like, and as soon as the lock clicked into place I felt deeply uncomfortable, almost panicked, in that tiny space. The small window, the walls that felt within reach were I to reach out my arms on either side of me; the ceiling above made me want to duck, as if it were lowering, as if the whole cell were closing in on me like a fist.

It is a prison requirement that at least three times a week, the Seg is visited by a doctor to ensure the occupants can cope with the conditions it imposes on them. However, during my time in Huntercombe, the cells in the Seg were often unoccupied. As David had pointed out when I first arrived, the types of prisoners serving their time there were less likely to cause trouble. Many were coming to the end of their sentences and just wanted to keep their heads down and stay out of trouble so as not to risk having time added to their sentence. There were others who would need to avoid trouble if they were in the process of trying to appeal against the decision to be deported.

So the Seg sometimes only had one or two cells occupied, but often they were all empty. Such a contrast to the Seg in Wormwood Scrubs, which was very much bigger and where the cells were usually all occupied. Visiting the Seg in the Scrubs could be quite challenging at times as some of the men were unpredictable and violent. Dirty protests were not uncommon and the fear of a surprise handful of faeces being thrown through a hatch was never far from my mind.

Regardless of whether the Seg was empty or not, however, I still had to attend and sign the logbook.

Prison rules. The days were thick with them.

On this particular day, however, after unlocking and locking again the door from Healthcare and walking along to the Seg, I heard a raucous noise which got louder as I unlocked the door at the other end of the corridor.

The two officers on duty were slumped in their chairs in the small office, looking totally exasperated, even though it was only eight thirty in the morning.

One of them, Joey, a big man with a belly that always seemed to be at war with the buttons of his uniform shirt, I knew from when I had first worked at Huntercombe in 2004.

'You don't want to be here, Doc,' he said, scratching idly at his belly. 'They're all very, very silly sods.'

The singing started again, and I realised that it was coming from four of the cells, the prisoners in each working together in harmony – just about – to form a chorus.

'What are they singing?' I asked.

The officer next to Joey sighed. 'It is a popular drinking song in Poland,' he said and I realised from his accent that he would know. 'My people sing it all the time. It is a very stupid song.'

With no enthusiasm whatsoever he started translating in time to the singing:

'Kuba drinks to his friend, Jacob; Jacob drinks to Michael; I drink to you, you drink to me. This is so lovely! Who won't drink because he is shy? He should be hit with two sticks. Whack-bang-whack-bang, yes he should be thrashed.'

We looked at one another for a moment.

'Well, that song took a turn,' said Joey.

'If you don't drink with us we'll beat you with sticks?' I asked.

The officer nodded. 'Two sticks. Whack-bang. It is a very stupid song.'

Joey smiled. 'They make good vodka in Poland.'

'Better vodka than songs,' his friend agreed.

'This is Jan, Doc,' said Joey. 'He's a right grump.'

'Only today,' said Jan. 'Because I have to sit here.'

'But why are they singing it?' I asked.

'They brewed up some hooch, didn't they?' said Joey, tapping away on his belly in time to the singing. 'Water, sugar, rotten fruit and a plastic bag kept somewhere warm. Job's done, and you've got yourself some time in the Seg where you can slowly, but ever so surely, make your way towards the worst hangover you've ever had.' He grinned. 'They're singing now, Doc, but they'll be crying in a bit.'

'And throwing up,' mumbled Jan. 'Do not forget that.'

Joey stopped smiling. 'You might be right there, I hadn't thought about that. Vomit really grosses me out. It's the sound more than anything. When it hits the tiles. Like a fat man slapping his wet belly.'

'I'd better go and see them, I suppose,' I said, 'and literally face the music!'

Jan nodded and got to his feet with a sigh. I sometimes felt sorry for the officers on duty in the Seg, as they often had to deal with some very disruptive people. On the other hand, if there was nobody in there, the shift must have been quite boring.

On that particular day, I think I'd rather have been bored. It would be better than being the audience of two for Poland's latest entry into the Inebriated Eurovision Song Contest.

'I'd stand back if I were you, Doc,' said Jan, as he tapped on the first cell door to announce our arrival before he unlocked it. 'It won't come as any surprise to know that they're a bit wild and unpredictable today. I think they're harmless enough, just pissed out of their stupid brains, but best to be on the safe side.'

Over the years of doing Seg rounds I have occasionally experienced prisoners spitting at people when the hatch in the door is opened, or worse, as I mentioned, throwing urine and faeces at whoever is on the other side of the door, so I was well aware of the unpredictable behaviour I might be subjected to.

There are also times, of course, when it's not safe to open the door or the hatch, and I have to have a conversation through the very small gap between the door and the doorframe.

Jan opened the door.

One of the singing voices rose in volume and I looked into the cell and saw an upside-down man poured across the bed and floor, arms raised to the air as if he was calling out his boozy love to a balconied Juliet. If she had the slightest taste she would empty a bucket of water on him.

'Are you okay?' I asked. He simply started singing louder, arms waving. 'He seems all right,' I sighed. 'For now.'

Jan stepped back, locking the door again, and moved on to the next cell. He opened the door and I peered in. The tipsy treble in our Polish choir was already starting to run out of steam, slumped in the corner of the cell. 'Fine,' I said. 'Obviously just need to keep an eye on them.'

Jan nodded as we backed out and closed the door.

'Mummy Jan will make sure his four naughty boys are tucked up safe and not about to choke.'

The occupant of the next cell could clearly hold his drink a little better than his compatriots. As the door opened he spread his arms wide to us as if greeting old friends.

'Hello,' I said. 'Just checking to see if you are all right?'

'All right?' he asked, briefly stopping singing. 'I am wonderful!'

'Well, that's good. Can't be all bad,' I said with a half-smile, nodding to Jan that he could close the door again.

When Jan opened the door of the fourth cell we were both presented with the sight of a large, completely naked man conducting the singing and prancing around the tiny space.

'Right,' I said, unfortunately no stranger to unbidden penises on duty. 'If he expects to conduct anything but a very small quartet with that then he's mistaken. But otherwise he's clearly fine.'

Jan laughed, nodded and closed the door. 'My countrymen are happy, they are awful and embarrassing and I wish they would shut up, but they are happy.'

I moved on to the final cell, knowing full well that this would, at least, be a break from the singalong. In cell five was a prisoner who was becoming something of a permanent fixture.

Jan opened the door and I stepped inside.

'The noise,' the cell's occupant said. 'I'm here to keep my

nose clean and they make me listen to that. How am I *not* going to kill anyone tonight?'

He was a huge man, utterly too big to be comfortable in the tiny Seg cell, which made it all the more surprising that it was his choice to be there.

Dima Tarr was a Hungarian man nearing the end of his sixteen-year sentence. He had a temper and, more to the point, seemed to attract more than his fair share of violence. He claimed that staying here in the Seg was the only way to guarantee he would be both safe and on track for his due release date.

His English was flawless, as, I had been informed, were several other languages he spoke. He had a small, perfectly formed grey beard and wore his long grey hair in a pony-tail. Everything about him was immaculate. Even there in that tiny space, his few belongings were placed with consideration and care. He had taken a room that would have looked cluttered simply by placing a pack of cards in it, and somehow made it feel pleasant.

Pride of place were his books, a neat pile of paperbacks of all different sorts. From crime thrillers to classics. I glanced at the book on top: it was a book called *Bone Machine* by Martyn Waites.

'It's not bad,' said Dima, seeing me looking. 'I know the author.'

'Oh, really?'

'He interviewed me a few times, you know ...' Dima grinned. 'Wanting to get material.'

'And I'm sure you were able to give him plenty,' I said. Dima was known to go on a fair bit. I never minded; he certainly had enough stories in him to fill a few pages.

He had been an armed robber – though he insisted that he *had* never, and *would* never have pulled the trigger. 'It's theatre, Doctor,' he said once. 'Only an amateur needs to pull his trigger. I don't need to shoot people, I just need them to *think* I could.' He had preyed solely on the extremely rich. 'Not because I'm Robin Hood,' he had joked once, 'but because I'm lazy and I am sensible. I am not going to risk being in a place like this unless it's worth it. When I step onto my stage, gun in hand and scary grin in place ... I want to be earning big!'

According to Dima – and his tales were sometimes as improbable as they were long – his career had seen him take fortunes from giants of business, heads of state and Hollywood actors. ('He cried like a baby, Doctor, the big action hero, the man they pay the big bucks to have the muscles and run through the explosions. He had wet cheeks and wet pants when I stepped onto his yacht. He offered me his wife if I would only spare him. I am pleased he is now divorced. What sort of person does that? Pig.')

He claimed – always with a wink – that he had plenty of money to look forward to once he got home. 'I look after my kids and they will one day look after me.'

'Now, honestly, Doctor,' he said, 'do you think they would tell me I have to stay here longer if I kill those four? I will be doing them a favour, yes?'

'Behave yourself, Dima,' I replied. 'Clearly you're doing all right?'

'I am always doing all right,' he replied. 'Though I need to see Asma again.'

'Asma the librarian? I asked.

'Yes, I need more good books to read. Always. I will always need more books. I have just read *The Beauty of Murder* by a woman called A.K. Benedict; it was very, very good and I need to know what else she has written. I need to read all the books by her.'

'Don't tell me,' said Jan. 'Tell the librarian.'

'It is not urgent for today,' he said. 'I cannot read good books while they sing. It's like trying to watch a beautiful film while someone dances in front of the screen. It is distracting.'

'I can imagine. I'll leave you to it, Dima.'

'Must you? At least while you're here I have a distraction. Did I ever tell you about the time I stole Tom Selleck's watch?'

'You're making it up.'

'Never. What about when I challenged the King of Sweden to a game of dominoes with his crown as the prize?'

'Don't be daft, Dima! Enough of your stories, I've got work to do.'

'You will regret it, Doctor, it's a fabulous story.'

'I'm sure.' I nodded at Jan and we backed out and Jan locked the door behind us.

'All good?' asked Joey, still slumped in his chair.

'All good,' I agreed, as I signed the logbook.

Suddenly code blue was called over the officers' radio and the doors to the Seg crashed open. It was Darren, the mental health nurse, who came running in.

'Quickly!' he said. 'It's Usama.'

'Usama?' I said. My heart felt as if it had stopped. Code blue. Usama. 'What's happened? What's he done?'

Darren shivered, pulling on his piercing, nervous. 'He's tried to hang himself.'

Chapter Thirteen

HMP HUNTERCOMBE
7 MARCH 2014

Code Blue.

As Darren and I ran towards Howard Wing and Usama's cell, I couldn't help but think back to when I'd last seen him. That distant look in his eyes, that need to thank me. Should I have seen something else? Should I have realised that this was a man who was close to the edge?

No. Usama had always been close, but should I have recognised him as someone who was slowly, irrevocably toppling over it? At least I knew that we were *all* looking out for him, so took some comfort in that. He was on an ACCT book more often than he was off it. Prisoners identified as being at risk of suicide or self-harm are put under the Assessment, Care in Custody and Teamwork process to keep a close watch on them.

But it is still so, so easy to blame yourself with hindsight, although deep down I knew that I couldn't help Usama in the way that he needed. I knew that I couldn't change the nightmare he was living in, however much I wanted to.

I had nothing to offer that could ever take away the total emptiness and feeling of desolation that he lived with every day.

People were running from all directions, knowing full well that someone's life was in the balance – that seconds could be all that might make a difference, all of us dreading what we might be faced with when we reached our destination.

Question after question flew through my head at a speed that matched my feet. But in my heart I knew that the blame for Usama's urge to die lay thousands of miles away and many months ago. The blame lay with a culture of violence and oppression, of brutal people-traffickers and a conflict in a distant country, not within the prison walls.

The only thing that mattered now was the need to save his life, even though there was a nagging and dreadful worry that he may not *want* to be saved. He had made the decision to end his life. Usama had wanted to die. He had realised – presumably – that between living with what had happened and not, he preferred to not. He wanted it all to stop. The hurting, the uncertainty, the pain. He wanted an end.

But it was really impossible to know what he thought, and every single person that day had a responsibility to try to save his life.

We ran down the long corridor towards Howard Wing. The people ahead of us had opened the gate and Officer Holland was waiting for everyone to pass through so that he could lock it again behind us, to save time, as clearly, right now, every second could make a difference.

'Straight down to the end, Doc,' he said as we ran past him. 'Last cell on the left.'

Not that we needed telling, as the door was open and a few people were gathered outside.

My heart was racing so fast when I got there that I could hardly breathe.

Would I find Usama dead? It just didn't bear thinking about. But to my total and overwhelming joy and relief I saw that Saroj, Rosemary and an officer were already performing CPR. The defibrillator pads were in place and he was alive. Usama was alive!

I offered to take over chest compressions to give one of them a break, as it is exhausting performing CPR. Rosemary nodded, so I stepped over her and then kneeled down next to her so that I could take over the next set of compressions.

Time seemed to evaporate, so I had no idea how long we had been working on him when the paramedics arrived and took over, much to our massive relief. When it was safe to move him, he was transferred onto a trolley and wheeled away, and soon was out of sight and on his way to hospital.

An eerie silence fell over the small gathering of people outside his cell, as everyone was left trying to absorb and reflect on the horror of what had happened.

It was then that I noticed a young officer who looked white with shock, and so upset I thought he was about to break down.

'Are you all right?' I asked.

'I found him,' he said. 'It was awful. I've never seen anything like it before. I thought he was dead. He had a torn strip of his sheet tied round his neck, and the other end was tied around the radiator. He was leaning forward, and I really thought he was gone. It was impossible to untie the knot and get him free, it... it just wouldn't loosen so I used my Fish knife. I didn't think that I'd be able to save him. I've never had to use it before and my hands were shaking as I tried to cut him free and when I did, he just slumped forward. It was so horrible ...'

His voice trailed off as he was clearly struggling to cope with the horror of what he had just been involved with.

I saw Pastor Clive among the small crowd of people, and realised that he was muttering a prayer under his breath.

'The pastor started the CPR,' said the officer. 'He's the one who helped me keep him alive until the nurses arrived.'

Pastor Clive had finished praying and he looked over towards me and gave a rather sad smile.

Anyone involved with the incident was invited to attend a debriefing with the governor, as is customary after being part of such a distressing and traumatising situation. It is a chance for people to share their feelings and support one another, but I didn't want to attend. At such times, and sadly there have been a few now, I need to be alone for a while to process my thoughts and find the strength to get back to work.

When I had finished for the day, instead of going straight home, I decided to go over to the craft centre.

I tapped on the door as I didn't have the right key for it, and was welcomed by an elderly officer I hadn't met before, with a kind and weathered face. He greeted me warmly and allowed me to wander round.

It was like entering another world, so far removed from the prison. It looked like an art classroom, white walls, shelves filled with brightly coloured objects, unfinished projects and paint-spattered books. On one table there were several models of human heads made out of twisted tissue paper in the process of being painted. On another there were unpainted wooden shapes, silhouettes of children's toys, gingerbread men star-jumping, racing horses caught mid-leap. At the head of the table there was a cuddly toy of a racoon, the black bands around its eyes turned into a robber's eye mask.

'It has become our logo,' said a voice behind me. I turned to see Bogdan Kolev, the young Bulgarian man whom I'd last seen being dragged out of my consultation room by officers.

'Mr Kolev?'

He looked sheepish. 'I shamed myself before,' he said. 'In your room. Please forgive me.' Then, without giving me time to reply, he reached forward and picked up the racoon. 'This, our logo. It is good, do you think?'

I nodded. 'Definitely appropriate.'

'If you want to buy one they are for sale. I will make a note of it and you can pay later? It would be good if you have children.'

'My boys are far too old for cuddly toys,' I said. 'But I will buy one for my friend's grandson. He will really love it, I'm sure.'

'We have lots of other things you may like,' Mr Kolev continued. 'Jewellery, maybe? There is a man from Romania, who makes very beautiful things. Or candles? You like candles?' He moved over to a shelf and picked up a pair of white candles in carved wooden holders. 'They smell of ...' he stopped to think then sniffed them. 'I do not remember. Is that jasmine? Or vanilla? Or something else?'

'I think it's jasmine. They are really lovely,' I said.

'It is good, the smell,' he agreed, nodding and putting the candles back on the shelf, immediately being distracted by something else. 'But look at all these beautiful decorations made from paper. A young Vietnamese man makes them and they are like little works of art.'

It was true, they were.

Mr Kolev was clearly so proud of all the items for sale that I didn't have the heart not to buy anything, and so put a little collection together. And then I realised why I was really there. 'Actually,' I said, 'there was something else I wanted too.'

*

I set off for home, but as I was driving my thoughts were soon invaded again by the prison and all the stories I had heard throughout the day. But most of all I thought of Usama. The memory of his face clung to me and refused to let go. Usama and Elias, two people in search of shelter. Hoping to find kindness.

It was a magical, cold and clear night, with a beautiful full moon and a mass of stars twinkling like little gems. When I arrived home, I was greeted by a welcoming smell of the meal my husband David was cooking, and the warmth and glow of a beautiful fire.

We talked briefly about what we had both done all day, and I mentioned Usama.

'He's hurting so much,' I said.

'Yes,' David agreed. 'But, thanks to everyone's efforts today, he's been given another chance. In time his pain will ease. It always does.' His wonderful voice of calm and reason was so reassuring. It had helped me so many, many times over my life when I was sad or anxious.

'Dinner will be ten minutes.' He turned to the oven and peered through the glass door. 'Probably.'

'I'm just going to get something out of the car,' I said.

I still had my big, warm overcoat on, and so, having put my new purchase in the corner of the garden, I stood quietly in the beautiful crisp night for a little while, mesmerised by the stars and the magnificent full moon.

The night was silent apart from the sound of the wind in the trees, and the faint scampering and twitching of animals in the open land around our garden. I hoped that, somewhere out there, something might need a home. Just as Usama had done.

No, not something. That's not what Usama had wanted. *Two* somethings. It had to be two.

I looked at the hedgehog house and began to cry.

Chapter Fourteen

HMP HUNTERCOMBE
April 2014

Tick tock, tick tock …

We're all born with clocks inside us. Forever counting down. Ticking away the years until puberty, the years within which we could still bear children, the years we might have left.

We try not to think about it, of course we do, and sometimes, in fact *most* of the time, you can't even hear the ticking. Because we're always surrounded by countdowns. The countdown until we start work or school, until we eat lunch, until our shifts are over, until we go to bed, until the morning alarm where we'll wake up and do it all over again. The countdowns to birthdays, to anniversaries, to Christmas.

Tick tock, tick tock.

The clocks are ticking all the time.

That year I could hear two in particular, all the time. The first was ticking down the months and weeks I had left at Huntercombe, the second was counting down the days Kofi Aboah had left to live.

'Morning, Doc!' Terry was in a particularly good mood that morning. Sipping from his dog's face mug I could imagine him as a jolly spaniel running through a field, tongue lolling, eyes wild. 'And isn't it a lovely one?'

'It is,' I agreed, showing him my pass.

The cold that had dogged winter had finally thawed into a delicious, golden spring. One of those Aprils where, if the low sun caught everything just right, it would look as if syrup had been poured across the world.

'How's things in the wild world of Healthcare?' he asked.

'Oh, you know, we manage by the skin of our teeth. Like everyone.'

'True enough,' Terry laughed. 'You know, every now and then, I think about that. About how, when I was a kid I looked forward to growing up and becoming all-knowing, completely in control, completely on top of absolutely everything.'

'And then you grow up.'

'And realise you're still just muddling through on a day-to-day basis. Annoying innit?'

'At least life is never boring.'

'Oh, I'd love boring, me. Just a brilliant slab of dull. A whole week of it. Nothing but staring at these four walls, dunking digestives in my tea and pretending I'll ever be able to solve *The Times* crossword. Bliss.'

*

Tick tock, tick tock, tick tock …

I sat in my room, working through the morning's patients. An elderly Korean gentleman and I spent an energetic five minutes miming the symptoms for an inflammatory bowel; I attended to a very severe flare-up of psoriasis suffered by a young man from Thailand; people from Afghanistan, Bali, Dubai, Lithuania and Pakistan told me how their returning to these countries after decades away would be, quite simply, the worst thing that could happen to them; and, finally, I shared a comfortable ten minutes with Habib Khan.

'You look tired,' he said, then put his hand to his mouth. 'Oh! That could sound rude, I do not mean it to.'

'Not rude at all, Habib,' I said. 'Are you ever? I *am* tired. It's been quite a morning and I'm not sleeping very well at the moment.'

'Bad sleep is the worst thing, is it not?' he said, nodding so vigorously I feared for his trapezius muscles. 'I used to have really bad bouts of it. You know what I did?'

'No, though I'll take any advice you have to offer.'

'I used to eat toast.'

'Ah.'

'Lots and lots of toast. A tower of toast. With all the Marmite I could find. Do you know, when the world ends and it comes time for the final books to be written and the final tallies struck, I think the main glory that this country will be blessed for is the invention of Marmite.'

'Not everyone would agree with you there.'

'Only the people with taste. When I die I wish to be

buried in a coffin filled with its unctuous brown glory. Or maybe clotted cream; I have yet to finalise my will.'

I smiled. 'Marmite would preserve you better.'

'I will be dug up in years to come, a perfectly preserved specimen lifted out of the yeasty swamp. Prehistoric Portly Pakistani, they'll put me in a museum.'

'An example of one of the funniest and nicest patients a doctor could have.'

'You flatter me doctor, but I do all I can to make you feel better after a hard morning.'

*

Tick tock, tick tock, tick tock …

Spring becomes summer and the golden light changes for a washed-out, watered-down world.

'And how are you feeling?' I asked Mr Wakabi.

He shrugged and sighed. 'I'm not gym-ready right now, I'll say that much.'

'You'll get there, I promise.'

From that initial consultation, a tiny bump that seemed most likely to be a tear from weight-lifting, Mr Wakabi had found himself moving from one urgent scan to another. Once a biopsy had been performed it was clear that the bump was nothing so benign as the result of keeping fit: he had spindle cell sarcoma, a malignant tumour. After the sarcoma was excised he underwent a course of chemotherapy and now, months later, he was battered but, thankfully, unbroken.

'I'm so glad I came to see you,' he said. 'I so nearly didn't, you know. So nearly.'

'But you did, and thankfully there's no reason that, moving forward, you won't make a full recovery. Your body's taken a bit of a pounding but you'll get over it. Promise.'

He nodded. 'I'll be back in the gym in no time, eh?'

'That's the spirit!'

*

Tick tock, tick tock, tick tock ...

'David!'

I jogged along the corridor to catch up with David Redhouse. He was walking in that usual, deceptively casual but terribly speedy way of his. Years working in prisons probably did that to people – always in a hurry, always trying to keep ahead of the next emergency.

'Doctor Brown.' He smiled but there was more than a hint of sadness hiding behind it. 'Can I guess what you're going to ask me?'

'No news?'

'At the moment it's still looking like the Early Release Scheme is going to be Mr Aboah's best bet.'

'But that's going to be too long!'

'At least another six months.'

I shook my head. 'At that rate I'll have left Huntercombe before he does.'

'Don't remind me,' said David. 'You'll be missed.'

I tried to smile but the thought of Kofi Aboah weighed too heavily. How was he supposed to endure that long?

*

Tick tock, tick tock, tick tock …

'It's okay, Doctor, I know how it looks.'

Kofi's leg was shaking, and my mind went right back to that very first consultation. The jittery leg, the sweating brow, a man trying to hold in all the pain.

'The swelling is getting bigger, yes.' There was little else I could say. 'And how are you doing with the pain?'

'The pills used to do it but now …' He tried to smile but it just looked like a dog baring its teeth, a defensive gesture of pain and fear. It was clear that the medication needed to be increased again

'I can increase the dose a bit more,' I said. 'I'm sure we can get it under control again. How did you get on when you went to the oncology clinic last week?'

He sighed. 'The doctor told me that he didn't think there is much more they can offer me, but he arranged some blood tests and said they would discuss me and my results at their next team meeting.'

'Oh, so I guess we just have to wait and see what they say. In the meantime, as I said, I'll increase the dose of your painkillers. We've got to try and keep on top of it

'Thank you, Doctor.' He looked at me and his eyes were

so sad. 'Please don't worry,' he said. 'I'll be all right. I'm not going anywhere.'

That's the problem, I thought. Then I realised he didn't mean it in the sense of leaving prison.

'I told you, Doctor,' he said, 'I'm going to see my family. Nothing's going to stop me. Don't worry about that.'

*

Tick tock, tick tock, tick tock ...

'Look at the state of *It*,' said Asma, holding up a battered copy of a Stephen King novel. 'I sometimes wonder if they read the books or try to make love to them.'

'Thank you for that image, Asma,' I said.

'Pleasure. I hope it gets you through the rest of your day.'

I walked over to the far corner of the small library where Usama was sitting at a table, writing.

'Hello, Usama,' I said. 'I hope I'm not interrupting?'

He looked up. I couldn't help but look at his throat, but was pleased to see that the faint scarring from the ligature had completely faded, and there was no mark left at all to remind him of that hateful day.

'Hello, Doctor,' he smiled. 'I have not seen you for a while. You are glad, no?'

'Well, Usama, I wouldn't put it quite like that. It's always a pleasure to see you, but I'm glad you haven't needed me.'

'Have you heard?' he asked. 'About my deportation?'

'No?' There was no reason anybody would tell me, of course; my purview began and ended with the prisoner's health.

'My lawyer has won. I do not have to go back to Syria.'

'That's wonderful!'

'The news of the fighting there is on the television every day, and in the newspapers … It is hard to send anyone back into that. It feels stupid, but I suppose I actually have reason to be grateful for how terrible it is back there. If it were just my home's thoughts on … well … ' He looked ashamed. 'Certain friendships.'

'Friendships that are none of their business, frankly,' I said, 'and certainly nothing to be ashamed of.'

He shrugged slightly and changed the subject. 'I am writing about it all.' He tapped the paper. 'He said it would be helpful and he was right, it makes things feel very different, to take it all out and put it on paper.'

'Who said? Darren, the mental health nurse?'

'No!' Usama laughed and I realised that was the first time I had ever heard him do that. 'Pastor Clive.'

'Oh! Have you been seeing a lot of him?'

'A bit. He believes in the wrong God, obviously, but other than that he's nice.'

I grinned. 'I like him, too. So, will you be moving on? Are they transferring you to another prison?'

'I'm due for release shortly, so they're going to let me finish my sentence here.'

'Well, that's good. I presume you'd rather stay here than have to start over somewhere else?'

'Yes, definitely. I've moved around enough for now.'

I looked down at the paper in front of him, row after row of neat marks, a life poured out. The difficult parts of his history put somewhere where they might be able to be shelved. That sounded healthy to me.

'Well, I'd better let you get back to it,' I said. 'You know where I am if you need me.'

'Thank you, Doctor.' He was already looking back at the paper in front of him, beginning to write. I imagined he had a lot to tell. I also imagined it would be heartbreaking to read.

*

Tick tock, tick tock, tick tock …

'Well, it's all right for some.' Rosemary smiled. 'Off you go again, eh?'

'Yes,' I agreed. 'Off I go again.'

I buttoned up my coat against the late autumn chill and gave Rosemary a hug. 'Keep them all in line for me,' I said. 'They'd be lost without you.'

'I know, I know … ' She laughed. 'How are you going to manage though?

'I'll muddle through somehow,' I said with a smile.

Walking out of Healthcare for the last time, boots hammering the hollow beneath us, I was wracked with the sense of unfinished business, as I had experienced so very many times in my life. So many stories I would never hear the end of. So many people I cared about who I would never see again.

But imagining Kofi Aboah still sitting in his cell while I stepped out into a chill November night, the swirls of crisp leaves circling around my feet, never to see him again or know the end of his story, felt too awful and made me feel so very sad.

Hadn't I promised that I would do everything I could to ensure he would see his family before he died? I'd been so determined to make the difference, to push it just that little bit further.

But instead …

*

Tick tock, tick tock, tick tock …

The phone rang. I answered.

'The date's confirmed,' said David Redhouse. 'Can you make it?'

He told me the date and, in truth, it didn't matter, there was no way I'd miss this. No way at all.

'How's he doing?' I asked, afraid to but how could I not?

'I'm amazed he's still with us. He's a very strong, very determined man.'

I was nodding, which was particularly pointless on the phone. 'He is. Very.'

'We'll see you then.'

*

Driving beneath the tree canopy, that dark, mulch tunnel that takes you away from the open skies and into the world of Huntercombe, I couldn't help but reflect back on the first time I'd returned there, unsure of the changes I would find, uncertain as to how I would fit in with the prison's new purpose. It was the same hard, frozen ground. Mud trails turned into preserved crime scene swirls by the frost.

I parked my car and found myself staggering cautiously across the icy ground just as I had done all that time ago, making a desperate beeline for a dirty snail trail of salted grit and safe footing.

'Now who can't stay away?' asked Terry as I walked in. Then his face became soft and gentle. 'I'm glad you could make it. It'll help, I think.'

'That's all I ever want,' I told him. 'To be of help.'

'I meant it'll help you,' he smiled. 'We all have ghosts, you know, the people we meet and who end up plugged into our lives. The people we take home with us at the end of the day.' He tapped his head. 'In here. And we never know how their stories pan out. They just vanish from our lives and we're left to wonder. Well, *hope*, really. This is your chance to get a bit of closure. It'll make all the difference, I'm telling you.'

'I can believe it,' I said, trying to fight back the tears.

He nodded again. 'I'll tell the boss you're here.'

After a couple of minutes, David appeared.

'Doctor Brown,' he said. 'Today's the day.'

'Finally.'

'Come through.'

He led me through to his office and sat me down at the meeting table. Again, the day was mirroring that first return visit.

'Would you like a cup of coffee?' he asked, the mirror still perfect.

'I'm fine,' I said, more to break the pattern than any other reason.

'He'll be ten minutes or so,' said David. 'I'd like to show you something while we wait, if you don't mind?'

'Of course not.'

He pulled over a laptop and cued up a video.

'Huntercombe Stories' announced a title card before a bulky Polish man greeted the camera and began to explain about his previous life, a life of drug use and theft. Cycles of addiction. Spells in prison. Then his time in Huntercombe, finding release in the gym and getting encouragement from the staff. He led classes, gained experience. Now he was working as a private trainer in Poland and running weight-lifting sessions in his local gym.

This was, of course, the project David had told me about when we were reunited here. His determination to record the success stories, to have a document of those men who had left there to find their efforts rewarded.

'Wonderful,' I said. 'It works really well.'

'The budget was a nightmare, wangling a local crew to handle the filming, but it's worth it. However many times you or I tell a prisoner they can change … Well, it's not worthless, of course not, but it's easier to ignore. If they hear it from someone who's been through the system. Someone who *really* knows.'

'It's got to have more weight,' I agreed. 'It's really inspiring.'

'I think so. Time will tell if I'm right!'

There was a knock on the door. I looked up to see Rosemary and Officer Holland. David jumped to his feet. 'Come in, all of you.'

I nodded at Rosemary who gave me a gentle smile as they filed in, Kofi Aboah between them.

He was so thin! His skin so pallid, the swelling in his neck so pronounced. His eyes were rheumy, his balance fragile. But here he was, beyond his time, still here, ready for his family.

'Doctor,' he said, his voice little more than a whisper. 'Nice to see you. You didn't have to come.'

'Of course, I did, Mr Aboah,' I replied. 'Of course, I did.'

There followed the practicalities. David running through the process, the trip to the airport. How Kofi would be placed on an aeroplane and then left – there was no need for him to be accompanied from that point on. As per Home Office legislation, authorities in Ghana had not – and would not – be informed that he had returned, that was a matter of confidentiality. He was handed a bank card.

'That,' said David, 'is the card to an account that holds the funds from your Facilitated Returns Scheme. There is £500 in there now, which you will be able to draw out in local funds on your return. In a month's time there will be a final payout of £250.'

Kofi nodded.

'Under these schemes,' David continued, 'you agree not to return to the UK within a period of five years.' He dashed the words off; he had to say them but we all knew they were meaningless.

David handed over forms for Kofi to sign and then, red tape done, he folded all the paperwork away and held out his hand for Kofi to shake.

'Mr Aboah, I wish you and your family the very best,' he said.

'Thank you, Governor,' Kofi replied, shaking David's hand.

He turned to me. 'Oh, never mind shaking hands,' I said and hugged him. He was so thin it felt as if I could feel every single bone. For the brief moment I held him all the memories of the times I had spent with him came flooding back and for the second time that day I fought hard to hold back the tears.

'Mr Holland?' David asked.

'Sir.' Officer Holland placed a gentle hand on Kofi's arm and he and Rosemary led him towards the door. Kofi stopped for a moment in the doorway and turned to face us.

'I shouldn't be here,' he said. 'I have lived beyond my time. In no small part down to your support. So thank you. My family thanks you.'

And with that he was gone.

*

Later and a letter drops through the letterbox from David. Enclosed is the photograph Kofi had always carried. Apparently he had left it in his cell with a little note for me. 'I suppose,' wrote David, 'he decided he no longer needed it and wanted you to remember him.'

I keep it in a drawer of letters and cards that I have received from prisoners over the years. It sits next to another that I printed off from an email. The second picture is similar to the first. The same house, the same family – all a bit older, a bit more weathered – the only difference is who else is there. Kofi Aboah, and although he was looking very thin and frail, he was more upright than I had ever seen him. His arms, his thin, thin arms, attempting to embrace the people he lived for.

I shouldn't be here.

That phrase keeps circling back round to me. Over and over again.

But I was. I was where I needed to be. And for all the

pain, the sleeplessness nights, the violence, the death and the tears, I wouldn't have it any other way.

For Kofi Aboah, for Usama, for Aaden, for Habib ... For every prisoner who had touched my heart and who in turn enhanced my life, for everyone who needed me ...

I was there.

Acknowledgements

As I was nearing completion of my third and final book, my world as I knew and loved it collapsed. My life changed forever when my beloved husband David died of a cancer so vicious that he was taken from me in less than four weeks. The man I have loved with all my heart and soul for over forty years is no longer by my side, and adjusting to life without him has been the hardest and saddest thing I have ever had to do. The deep and agonising pain of grief is overwhelming and ever present, and I feel utterly broken. There is no doubt that the belief David had in me shaped my life, and no words can ever adequately express my love for him, and the sadness I feel since losing him. This book is dedicated to him, as he encouraged me to tell my story. Unlike me, he thought that it should be told. *The Prison Doctor* books would never have been written if it were not for him. During his short and savage illness, David was lucky enough to be looked after by some truly remarkable people in Stoke Mandeville Hospital to whom I will be forever grateful. The care he received was outstanding, and the kindness and compassion shown to me was beyond anything I have ever experienced before. Hospital staff, many of whose names I never knew, helped me through the darkest and saddest time of my life. They hugged me when I so desperately needed to be hugged. My heartfelt love and thanks to every single person who cared for David during the last weeks of his life, from the porter in A&E who wheeled him away from me when he first arrived, to the magnificent team in ITU where he died. You will never know the impact your kindness has had, and will always have, on my life.

My thanks to Guy Adams for helping me to write this book, and for the love and support he and his wife have shown me since losing David.

Also, to my agent and now, I hope, lifelong friend Susan Smith of MBA Literary Agents for her enduring belief in me.

To all the team at Harper Collins, especially my editors Kate Fox and Nira Begum for their encouragement and guidance.

Thanks also to all the wonderful people who have supported me through my grief. It is not possible to mention all by name as the list would fill another book.

Of special note, however, are my beloved sons, Rob and Charlie, who share my agony but give me a reason to live. They enhanced David's life with their love for him and with the incredible sense of humour they shared. He loved you both so very much and was so proud of you for being the truly wonderful people that you are.

My dearest sister Laurie and brother-in-law Nick for nurturing me with love, immense kindness and cake.

David's sisters Ros and Viv, and brother-in-law Juan, for managing to cheer me up when I thought it was impossible to do so.

Thanks to James and Tony of Legacy Funeral Services who were there for me in my hour of desperate need the night David died. I will be forever grateful to you for your ongoing kindness, friendship and love.

Thanks also to Joe Hage, Sarah Haynes and Adam Bates for the kindness, friendship and generosity you have shown me over the past year. I am so grateful to you all.

My love and thanks to Tony and Sally Mack, and to Roger and Jan Motson for the joy they brought to David's life by sharing their love of sailing with him. Also to Haley Murch, one of the kindest people I know.

Finally, my thanks to my beautiful and incredible friend Vanessa and her husband Bernard for taking me under their wing and loving me as if I were part of their extraordinary family. What a privilege!

I honestly don't know how I would have got through the past six months without all these magnificent people. Thank you, all of you, for helping me to somehow survive the desolation of grief.

And lastly, 'According to our strength of character and our clarity of vision, we will endure, we will succeed, we will have contributed something to make life where we were and as we lived it, better, brighter and more beautiful.' (Frank Lloyd Wright)

Thank you, David, with all my heart, for making my life better, brighter and more beautiful than it could ever have been without you in it. I long to be with you again.

ONE PLACE. MANY STORIES

Bold, innovative and
empowering publishing.

FOLLOW US ON:

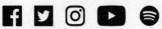

@HQStories